Get Out of Your Head

Be in Control of Your Life.
Break Free From Self-Limiting
Habits and Fear

Wallace Port

advice. The content within this book has been derived from various sources. Please consult a licensed professional before attempting any techniques outlined in this book.

By reading this document, the reader agrees that under no circumstances is the author responsible for any losses, direct or indirect, that are incurred as a result of the use of the information contained within this document, including, but not limited to, errors, omissions, or inaccuracies.

Table of Contents

"I suffer from low self-esteem. I had horrible self-esteem growing up. You really have to save yourself because the critic within you will eat you up. It's not the outside world — it's your interior life, that critic within you, that you have to silence."
~ Iman

Introduction

Would you believe that according to a news report several years ago, as many as 85% of Americans suffer from low self-esteem? This figure accounts for millions of individuals. People you possibly drive past, walk by, work with, commute with, or maybe even live with. Having picked up this book, I am almost certain that you are one of them, you live with one of them, or you know one of them. This book will assist you in understanding them better and perhaps discovering new ways of working with them.

If you happen to be experiencing any of the following, then you may have a self-esteem problem:

- "I'm sorry" is part of your everyday vocabulary.
- You battle establishing work or personal boundaries.
- You struggle to voice your opinion at crucial times.
- You believe in going with the flow rather than rocking the boat.
- You feel guilty about wanting more than you have.

- You go out of your way to be recognized and needed by others.
- You have negative beliefs concerning your body image.
- You prefer others making your choices for you.
- Your internal dialogue is harsh and unforgiving.
- Your own wants take second place to the needs of others.
- Your self-beliefs are mostly negative.

These are just some of the topics we'll cover in *Get Out of Your Head: Be in Control of Your Life. Break Free From Self-Limiting Habits and Fear.* In addition to these, we will break down what self-esteem is and why it is so important to your success or failure. We will also discuss things like why we feel we need to be validated in everything we do. This behavior can lead to personal defeat and self-limiting habits, which is what we are trying to overcome.

We will all go through times in our lives when our self-esteem and self-confidence are tested to the limits. This is what makes knowledge on how to handle each of these situations so important to have at your disposal. If you take just one valuable lesson away from this book, then I will have done my job. Naturally, I sincerely hope that there will be a host of valuable information that you find useful in the pages that follow, like golden nuggets of wisdom to be used whenever necessary.

There may be parts of this book that you may feel are too harsh or too direct in the way they are communicated. This is purely for your benefit. There are times when we are all faced with a bitter pill that we need to swallow. Hopefully, you will keep reading on and push past these "difficult to hear" sections because every piece of information in this book has been carefully selected especially with you in mind.

The information contained in the pages that follow does not follow a linear pattern. Instead of trying to digest these pages all at once, you may need to come back to individual chapters time and time again, and that is okay. Grab a notebook to write down things that strike you as important, or have a highlighter next to you for certain sections that you would like to remember. This is your personal guide for how to *Get Out of Your Head: Be in Control of Your Life. Break Free From Self-Limiting Habits and Fear.*

This book aims to provide you with actionable exercises and real solutions to turn down the volume to control your inner critic. It is here to help you work through your current belief system to identify fatal flaws and correct them.

Please understand that there is no pattern when it comes to being weighed down with these negative, self-defeating voices either. That voice inside your head is not asking for your permission to be there. The reason why it is there in the first place is that you have given it permission to be there. Don't believe me? Read on…

To be honest with you, the nagging little voice inside your head telling you that you are not good enough has no respect for people. It does not care what your bank balance looks like, where you come from, what your age is, or even your ethnicity.

Low self-esteem is like a cancer that needs to be cut out at the root to deal with it effectively and efficiently. Without physically doing everything in your power to get over it, you will constantly be facing those nagging voices in your head; you know the ones I am referring to.

As part of *Get Out of Your Head: Be in Control of Your Life. Break Free From Self-Limiting Habits and Fear,* we will take a deep dive into what causes these voices in our heads that drag us down constantly, making us feel like crap every day.

We will discover why this inner critic seems to hold so much power over us, preventing us from moving forward and being able to live the life that we want to live. We will explore our current lifestyle habits to determine whether any of these are presently causing us harm and adding to our low self-esteem.

One of the final causes we will investigate is that fatal flaw known as fear.

Once we have discussed each of these as reasons that are preventing us from moving forward toward the dreams, goals, and life that we know we deserve and are capable of, we will discuss what we can do about each of these points.

The main objective of *Get Out of Your Head: Be in Control of Your Life. Break Free From Self-Limiting Habits and Fear* is to make you realize that you hold the power to free yourself from these debilitating behaviors. You can change the trajectory of your life simply by making several small changes to your life.

This is not to say that your life will change instantaneously and overnight! Nothing ever does. What it is saying is that by working consistently and making incremental changes to the way you do things daily, you can develop a positive, healthy lifestyle and habits to benefit you in the long run.

We will consider the ultimate cost of low self-esteem, self-limiting habits, and fear in your life. How are these holding you back right now in various areas of your life? Because they are, whether you are ready to admit to it or not.

The tentacles of fear have far-reaching negative consequences and often squeeze every ounce of enthusiasm out of you, preventing you from even stepping out of your comfort zone. Instead, they keep you paralyzed in the moment, immobilized, and stuck in a rut.

We will also discuss all the emotions that come with each of these negative habits. Often, these include things like doubt, lack of self-confidence, and uncertainty, all of which are keeping you stuck in this moment. Many of these happen on a subconscious level, and before you can work through them, you need to be able to identify them.

Some of the things we will consider are the repercussions and negative impact that this inner critic and voice in your head can have in your life. By finding alternative ways of dealing with this inner critic, you may find the inner strength and tenacity you knew you had inside you all along. It is all about you learning how to get this inner critic under your control rather than the other way around.

In each of the chapters that follow, we will help you find alternative ways to gain that much-needed self-confidence, breaking out of your shell. The discipline that you need to move beyond the voices in your head and the voices of the world is within reach. All you need to do is believe. You need to believe in yourself and your ability to change whatever you set your mind to.

According to Mark Twain, "A habit cannot be tossed out the window; it must be coaxed down the stairs a step at a time."

Let's dive right in and discover where most of these voices come from.

Chapter 1:

Understanding Inner

Voices

"It's not what you say out of your mouth that determines your life;
it's what you whisper to yourself that has the most power."
~ Robert Kiyosaki

Whether we are happy to admit to it or not, we each have voices in our heads that we have internalized, and we allow them to show up uninvited, unannounced, and often at the most inconvenient times in our lives. So, where do these voices come from, and what makes them potentially bad? After all, some of the voices could be quite comforting and encouraging. Well, these positive voices are not the ones we are focusing on throughout this book. Instead, we are going to focus on the negative ones with the goal to replace each of the negative voices you're currently experiencing with positive ones.

Changing the Narrative

To replace our negative thoughts with positive ones, we have to be willing to make some changes. According to Gary John Bishop in his book, *Unf*ck Yourself: Get out of your head and into your life*, there are two specific trains of thought when it comes to deciding to make changes in your life. The first is by being 'willing' to do whatever it takes. This would refer to being prepared to get up early to exercise rather than sleeping in or hitting that snooze button.

The second way of looking at things we need to change in our lives is by being 'unwilling.' Bishop doesn't mean that you're simply unwilling to do whatever it takes; instead, he refers to this as being completely resolute that you are unwilling to continue on the same path that you've possibly been on for ages. You're unwilling to keep settling for the kind of life that you have at present.

For both, the same kind of internal resolution is what is necessary to pull off these changes and make your life situation better than what you are experiencing now. The question you then have to answer is: Are you willing (Gary John Bishop, 2017)?

What Do You Really Want?

Aligned with the above resolve is having a clear understanding of what you want and don't want. After all, if you don't know what you want, how can you be willing to change anything? Say you are looking to earn more money than what you are currently earning. Whether you believe so or not, this is much easier for you to accomplish than what you think. What you need to decide is what you are prepared to either give up or sacrifice to accomplish whatever it is that you've determined is a worthwhile goal or objective.

If you believe that more money is going to make a difference in your life, then you need to be prepared to make the equivalent sacrifice to achieve this objective. In this instance, it will more than likely require a time sacrifice. Are you prepared to spend at least another 60 to 80 hours a month working to earn the kind of income you want to be earning?

However, if you want to spend more time with your family, then this is not going to be the solution you're looking for. You will need to be certain that your desires are closely aligned with whatever it is that you are prepared to sacrifice in response to what you genuinely want.

What Are You Prepared to Sacrifice?

If you're not prepared to sacrifice anything, then that's also okay. You just need to be happy or okay with the outcome of your life as it currently stands. You cannot hold anyone else accountable or responsible for the situation that you're experiencing in your life if you aren't prepared to do something to shift the outcome. This could apply to anything from receiving a promotion at work, earning more money, becoming physically fit, or losing weight.

Please understand that it's okay not to want the same things as everyone else around you. Can you imagine how boring the world would be if each of us were the same? If we each aspired for the same goals, level of education, relationship status, financial status–I think you understand what I'm getting at.

Of course, if you are unwilling to put in the time, effort, and energy to change, don't throw a fit when everything remains the same. If you don't want to sacrifice anything, then you can't experience receiving a reward in return. The short version of this is that you get what you work for.

Be prepared to admit to yourself that you are either willing to do the work and make the sacrifice to accomplish whatever goals you determine to be worthy and worthwhile or move on with other things that you are willing to do.

Winning and Losing

Here's a bit of a mind-bender: You need to recognize that you win even when you lose. Stop and read this sentence again. Yes, you read it correctly the first time. If you want that promotion at work, you must already know and accept that it's going to come with a whole lot of added responsibilities, particularly if it is a promotion with a title. It's going to come with longer hours or taking work home. Although you may have all the additional work and responsibilities that may require you to give up some of your personal time, you are still winning personally because of the promotion. Now, had you not received the promotion at work, you would still have an opportunity to win. You may be thinking that this doesn't make any sense at all. Even through defeat, you have an opportunity to learn something new about yourself. It will give you the chance to identify where you went wrong so you can fix it. It gives you the chance of becoming a better individual.

This doesn't only have to happen in terms of tangible things; it can also happen as part of the relationships we have with others. Just when you believe that everything is going well in a relationship, all of a sudden, it backfires horribly. You may be looking for answers in all the wrong places instead of trying to identify what went wrong and where and then trying your best to fix it.

I'm going to make another statement that you may not initially like or agree with. You attract exactly what it is that you put out there. What you may initially recognize as winning could easily turn destructive. This is by grand design. We attract into our lives exactly what we want. When our relationships fail, it's because of things like doubt creeping into our minds. This self-destruction mechanism comes into play because we attract it into our lives on a subconscious level.

Law of Attraction at Work

When it comes to relationships, we attract the same type of energy that we are putting out there. A lot of this is happening on a subconscious level, and we aren't even aware of it.

These all start with something simple like the thought "I'm so ugly that nobody out there will ever love me!" Guess what? That's exactly what happens because that is what you are attracting to your life.

But because this is subconscious, you don't even realize that many of these thoughts have been so deeply imprinted on who you are. This is the Law of Attraction happening at its simplest possible level. You keep thinking or telling yourself these things, and they are exactly what the universe is about to dish up and serve you!

So, where do all these thoughts come from? Childhood, parents, teachers, peers, siblings, and even social media—you're surrounded by images of perfection that you're trying to be like, when in reality, you are a unique individual. You don't need to try and become another version of someone else. This is probably one of the most difficult lessons for us to realize because we are always subconsciously measuring ourselves against everyone else out there.

To combat this need to compare ourselves, let's take a look at where we got these internal beliefs in the first place.

Internalizations

This subconscious belief system comes from experiences that you've internalized from a young age thanks to things that you were exposed to as a young child or teenager. These beliefs are often cemented by those that we trust the most.

By this, I'm referring to well-intentioned parents who may have implemented a strict form of parenting. It could be a result of parents who were fighting with each other consistently and then took that pressure out on you. Maybe it was a teacher who berated and belittled you in front of your class because there was something you never understood or you happened to make a foolish error. Often, peer pressure can also result in multiple negative subconscious belief systems.

What I mean by negative subconscious belief systems is that by the time you are an adult and possibly in a position where you need to begin making decisions and judgment calls for yourself, your belief system has already been negatively influenced. Because beliefs are formed at a young age, they will influence your decisions, actions, and life moving forward.

What Are Your True Beliefs?

Of course, you can't change your beliefs if you don't know what they are. You will need to complete an in-depth self-analysis to discover what your true beliefs are and what's holding you back and preventing you from moving forward in your life.

As part of this in-depth analysis, you can begin asking yourself some of these more difficult questions:

- Are your current beliefs limiting or liberating?
- Do they make you feel frustrated or fulfilled?
- Are these beliefs currently holding you back, or are they propelling you toward the goals that you have identified as being worth fighting for?

Whatever you are choosing to believe about yourself is what is keeping you stuck in your current pattern. Maybe you are held back by fear or other negative emotions like doubt, anger, frustration, self-loathing, and a defeatist attitude. As part of your belief system, are you functioning on autopilot most of the time? Many of us fall into this habit so easily that it is difficult to even identify that we are actually doing it.

Sleepwalking Through Life

Here are some seriously shocking statistics: Stem cell scientist, DNA specialist, and author of *The Biology of Belief: Unleashing the power of consciousness, matter & miracles* Bruce Lipton asserts that as much as 95% of everything we do is done while functioning subconsciously or on autopilot so to speak.

Think about driving your children to school every day or going to the grocery. How many times have you arrived at your destination or arrived back home without having any memory of the route you took or how you got there? I know that I can certainly own up to experiencing this on way too many occasions.

This is often where we feel as though we are sleepwalking through our own lives. We need to be able to move the subconscious into the conscious. This is where we are fully present in the moment rather than doing things automatically (Lipton, 2005/2016).

Whatever you are focusing on most of the time on a subconscious level is what your brain is actively working toward. You may not realize that when you are intently focused on something on a subconscious level, you can turn this into your reality. The 'reality' you are currently experiencing is a direct result of your belief system that you have internalized subconsciously.

We don't really have too much control over where our subconscious thoughts are going. We need to try and switch it up a bit to become more self-aware of what thoughts we are processing rather than just being satisfied to listen to what our inner critic is telling us.

Inner Guide Versus Inner Critic

Let's not become confused with the voices that are from your inner critic and your inner guidance system. How can you even tell them apart? It's quite simple. Your inner guidance system will always tend to be softer; gentler; and encourage you to do more, be more, push harder, keep going, and not give up. This is the voice we can listen to and feel good about ourselves. Most of the time, it will encourage us to do our best and become the best version of ourselves we can be.

In contrast, the inner critic is going to tell you all the things that you can't do. It will try and make you feel lost and alone, like a fraud or a failure, just because that's what it's been programmed to do for all the years it's been around.

The two types of voices are completely different and serve different purposes in your life. You will easily be able to tell the difference between your inner critic and your inner guidance system by the topic of "inner conversation." This is the subject matter that your inner critic chooses to send in your internal direction.

There are various inner critics, and none of them are good. Some of these are as follows:

- The nagging inner critic, which is responsible for never keeping quiet and complains about everything. It is this inner critic that will keep tugging and tugging at something until it unravels.
- The questioning inner critic questions and analyzes everything to death. Every decision or action is played repeatedly as though on an endless loop.
- The egocentric inner critic could be based on your conscience. It is likely to play on your conscience much in the same way the questioning inner critic operates, except it targets your conscience instead.
- The judgmental inner critic cannot prevent itself from offering up loud (and often unrealistic) judgments about a person.

Each of these inner critics is aimed at derailing our lives.

To define more clearly what an inner critic is, keep in mind that it will always be criticizing harshly and prone to judging you for every action you may have made or failed to make. Our inner critic can prevent us from acting by making us feel like we are less than adequate or unworthy.

Imagine, for example, that you have been selected to be part of a project in your workplace. Some of the initial internal dialogue experienced from your inner critic may resemble the following statements:

- Why do they want you to be part of this team?
- You know you're going to end up failing hopelessly, don't you?
- What if you can't complete the project on time?
- You are the weakest link out of everyone else on the team.
- Maybe it's better to quit while you're ahead rather than drag everyone else down with you.
- Joe is so much better at this than you are; why didn't they just assign him?

You get the picture. This list can go on and on, and that voice in your head can continue pulling out all the stops to make you feel like crap to the point where you are ready to throw the towel in or you end up procrastinating when you could physically work on the assignment given to you.

The way you can tell this is your inner critic is because everything that you think and feel about yourself is negative. Criticism always seems to focus on the negative. It is focused on dragging you down rather than building you up (which is part of the reason why it is not a good idea). Another problem with having a harsh inner critic is that it can mess with the condition of your self-esteem, which has a knock-on effect when it comes to your physical, emotional, and mental well-being.

Those who constantly struggle with an overactive inner critic can find themselves completely paralyzed by fear. This is not the type of fear that you are in physical or mortal danger, but it can have similar effects in keeping you stuck in the moment. It is this fear that threatens to debilitate us, keeping us paralyzed in the present.

What Causes Inner Critics?

Various things could have caused your inner critic to become so vocal in your life. Most of these are linked with situations that happened in childhood. While you may not realize it, a lot of what you think about as an adult has directly been shaped by the way you were treated as a child. The voices and language you heard as a child could have been negatively influenced by parents, teachers, siblings, and even peers.

Comments that were directed at you or you happened to be exposed to have led to the incessant background chatter that seems to be consuming your brain constantly. It is these voices that have molded and shaped who you have chosen to become. You may not even realize that you are hanging on to things from the past that are creating this inner talk and inner critic.

You may have been told many things that were unkind or even cruel as a child, and this is what has been carried through into adulthood. Typical examples of this are things such as:

- He's not very bright, is he?
- Her hair is all frizzy, and that just makes her look weird.
- Why are you still eating? You're so fat already.
- Don't bother entering; you're no good anyway.

Each of the above expressions can crush someone's self-confidence and self-esteem completely as a child, let alone as an adult. Without the correct tools to be able to direct you out of this way of thinking, you are likely to get stuck with these debilitating thought patterns for the rest of your life.

The sad part is that people often say things in frustration or anger not meaning anyone any harm, but once the words have been said, it is not possible to get them back, no matter how hard they try.

What is really disconcerting is that most people don't understand the amount of power they actually give away when they choose to listen to their inner critic and the ultimate effect that it can have on their lives holistically. One of the main areas that feel the impact of a harsh inner critic is our self-esteem.

Self-Esteem

Let's take a brief look at what self-esteem looks like from the outside. If you had to try and define self-esteem, the closest you would get to it would be self-estimate. What do we think and feel about ourselves? How do we think we compare to the rest of the world? When we look at it like this, it is laughable that we would want to even compare ourselves with our neighbors, let alone the rest of the world.

Self-esteem can be divided into two distinct groups, either healthy or unhealthy self-esteem or self-estimate. A healthy self-estimate is where we feel comfortable in our own skin. Believe it or not, there are far more individuals out there who fall on the opposite end of the spectrum and suffer from low self-esteem instead.

In addition to low self-esteem, there's another type of self-esteem that can really sabotage us if we are not careful. Unhealthy self-esteem is where you are on the verge of being unable to function because you think so little of yourself. You are constantly weighed down and stressed by how not only others perceive you but also your inner critic, which is there telling you that you're unacceptable.

The relationship that we have with our self-esteem is then linked to our self-confidence. How do we feel about ourselves out in the world?

Can you see how there could be a direct correlation between these two? You need to be able to understand this correlation before you can even begin to do anything about it. The most important thing is remaining unstuck to be able to move forward in the world and with your life.

One of the most pertinent questions when it comes to all the above seems to be why we believe it necessary to choose to listen to these voices in our heads. Stop and re-read this sentence again! There it is, the word 'choose.' We forget that we have full control over ourselves, our lives, the thoughts we have, and what we choose to believe.

Part of the reason for choosing to listen to the voices in our heads is because they are always there. If you think about it, going back to your earliest recollection, you will always recall having the constant companionship of voices in your head. In many instances, they are not always negative. These are not the voices that we are worried about in this book.

We are more concerned with those that are destructive. The ones that we allow to take center stage too often in our lives rather than relegating them to an understudy role where they are not even on the stage that is our mind. But none of that answers why we choose to listen to them. There is an answer, though, and it is validation.

Validation

We listen to them because we have been programmed to need every thought and action validated. What do I mean by this? Remember when you were still a young child or in grade school? Whenever you managed to complete a task successfully, you sought out your parents, guardians, or teacher for their validation and approval. You needed their approval to know that the choices and decisions you had made were correct.

Now though, as an adult, you should no longer be worried about the validation and approval of others. The only person's approval and validation you should need is your own. However, that is rarely the case. Many of us still find ourselves looking for external validation.

Waiting for the approval of someone else shows that you want to work according to their experience or standard of excellence rather than worrying about your own quality of work yourself. You would rather let someone dictate their conditions to you than remain free to choose to act on your own internal instincts. By this, I am referring to that gut instinct that we all possess. We should all be able to tell right from wrong simply by relying on our internal moral compass.

Moral Compass

Let me ask you this: Do you know when you have made a mistake? Sure, you do. That is all part of your moral compass or your internal code of conduct. These are the things that you do and behaviors you are happy to live your life by. They will determine things like whether you are honest and ethical in your dealings with those around you.

Your moral compass guides you in each decision you make, or it should. When you choose to live your life according to someone else's moral compass or value system, all you are going to get in return is a hollow and empty sensation. The reason for this is that it is not part of who you are. No matter how good their value system may be, it has not been internalized as your own. This, once again, leads to your inner critic having full reign over the situation, leaving you feeling lousy and defeated.

The nagging voices in your head can make you feel less than adequate, keeping you stuck in the moment because you believe them. They can play a major role in being able to shape who you believe you are as well as your identity out in the world.

The Effect of the Inner Critic

Your inner critic voice is the one that's telling you all the things you don't want to hear because you know that they are only going to hold you back. It is messing with your level of self-esteem and self-confidence. Some can fool the world by appearing to be well adjusted, successful, and have it all together on the outside. This, however, may just be a façade, a mask that is there for the convenience of society. Deep down, they may be feeling unsure of themselves and unable to control all the voices screaming at them internally.

By listening to these voices, you often second-guess yourself and experience deep-seated emotions such as guilt and shame. These negative emotions often develop into not just inner criticism but self-criticism as well. This inner critic doesn't happen overnight; instead, it can be years and years of negative influences from those nagging voices that never seem to stop their never-ending chattering in our heads.

Some people may believe that they are experiencing auditory hallucinations whenever they hear these voices. This is certainly not the case as has been confirmed by psychologists and other mental health practitioners. These thoughts often encourage us to act against our own best interests. This is what results in self-sabotage and destructive behavior.

We're imagining each of these different voices, and they're all telling us different things. Other characteristics that these inner, self-critical voices have are that they coax us on to behave in ways that are out of the ordinary and can prove to be harmful to us. We often spend hours and hours of precious time ruminating over nothing more than destructive thinking.

You can easily become stuck in the moment if you believe what these voices are telling you about yourself. You are 'stuck' because of the negative voices and belief systems you have in your head. These voices and this belief system are preventing you from moving forward; they are causing you to question your own abilities, and so rather than doing something about it, you keep second-guessing every move that you make.

You keep yourself from moving forward purely out of fear. The fear that you won't be accepted; fear that you are likely to mess up because you're just not good enough; fear of failure; fear of not making the grade;

fear of not meeting targets; fear of not being a good enough partner, spouse, parent, friend; and so the list goes on and on.

You may be wondering how a couple of voices in your head can derail your life, preventing you from moving forward and living your best life possible. The truth is that these voices can and do impact almost every aspect of our lives. And it's not just our personal lives, or our business lives, or our careers. They can derail us completely to the point where we become so stressed out and full of anxiety that we withdraw from everything and everyone around us completely.

These negative thoughts undermine any positive thoughts you may have about yourself. Instead of that soothing, positive, soft voice that encourages you to try a little harder because with a little more effort you know you can get there, the voices you hear are much more abrupt, harsh, and unfriendly. They're judgmental, filled with self-loathing, and often pass this judgment and self-loathing on to others.

These are the voices telling you to give up on your goals and your dreams because there's no way you're ever going to achieve them. They will confirm in your ear that you're the misfit and the loser who doesn't get to live the good life. As a result, you may decide to pull away from any form of goal setting or work toward achieving something worthwhile, even for a short time.

Another influence that these critical voices can have on a person is to simply withdraw from the world. The long-term effects are that you doubt your own abilities.

In this chapter, we have covered a great deal of information with regard to what your inner critic is, the difference between your inner critic versus your inner guide, and how to tell them apart. We have also discussed ways that your inner critic has the ability to negatively influence a great many parts of your life. In the next chapter, we will consider ways that your inner critic can contribute toward feelings of failure.

Chapter 2:

Your Inner Critic and

Failure

"What you tell yourself every day will either lift you up or tear you down."
~ Athena Laz

When choosing to listen to your inner critic instead of the voice of reason, you give your power away. You allow others to dictate what you are experiencing, and this holds you back and keeps you stuck. You choose to accept what each of these critics is telling you to be true, thereby limiting your progress.

This inner critic isn't just found within you, though. We all have one, and at some point, we have all listened to it.

We All Have an Inner Critic

Many of us don't even realize that we have an inner critic. We hear it in our heads and assume that it's our voice of reason rather than one of destruction. What's even worse than believing that it belongs to us is that it seems to shine a bright light onto each of our faults.

Each time it appears, it seems to be more and more believable. We believe that our life is a mess, that we are unable to make rational decisions, that whatever we do is likely to turn out a disaster just as much as our current life is a disaster. What we aren't realizing, though, is that we're creating our own enemy within. We listen to everything these voices in our heads say and live on tenterhooks by believing whatever the voices tell us.

Where Do They Come From?

What we don't realize is that these voices aren't our rational side; they're an entire community that has gathered to form an anti-fan club around us. They can easily be recognized because they're negative and condescending, filled with harsh judgments and a lack of self-belief. They will sabotage us in any way they can to prevent us from achieving our goals.

They often turn the volume up just enough to drown out anything constructive you may be thinking, and all you're left with are loud critics screaming at you from every direction. Whenever you're faced with them, accept them for who they are, and try to move on.

Are You Your Worst Enemy?

There's an adage that says, "You are your own worst enemy." In this instance, we could say, "You are your own worst critic." Discovering creative ways of dealing with these voices is what you need to look for. There are ways to reduce the volume to silence them, which we will discuss in greater detail as we get into this book. Let's just say that while we all need to be able to discipline ourselves and push ourselves to accomplish our goals, we don't necessarily need to go about it in the harsh way that our inner critic often does.

Trying to understand what your critic is can be a conundrum. So, what is it exactly? It's the voice that tells you that you're a failure, that you cannot possibly achieve something, that people aren't interested in you, that you don't have the talents to complete a specific project. In a word, it is going to tell you everything that you don't need to hear. Does this mean that whatever it is telling you is true? Definitely not!

You may not even know where these inner critics come from. Most of them stem from incidents that occurred when you were young, like when a teacher called you out in front of the class, or moments later in life where you were placed on the spot or failed horribly. How did you feel at the time? Like a loser? Like you couldn't accomplish what was possibly a simple assignment? These experiences throughout our lives leave us struggling when it comes to trying to calm our inner critic.

Failing produces a sense of doubt and a lack of confidence in yourself and your ability to succeed. It makes you think you will fail again, which seems to suggest a fatal flaw in your character and be a barrier toward success. This is so far from the truth. Anyone who understands how goals and success work will be able to understand that to achieve anything in life, we need to learn from our mistakes.

Failure Allows for Learning

If we think that we will go through life without making any mistakes, then we are confused about the way life works. Even as small children, we first need to learn the basics, like raising our heads on our own, balancing as we learn to sit, mastering how to crawl before we can walk, and finally learning to run. Imagine if all of this happened automatically without any mistakes? Do you think that we could ever be resilient or tenacious without learning some of these basic life skills?

We need to be able to fail to learn the lessons that will allow us to grow and develop into contributing members of society. These lessons begin at birth and continue throughout our lives. It may sound cliché, but there's no such thing as a free ride through life. One of the greatest lessons to learn when it comes to this is that failing is going to happen to all of us, and when it does, we need to be open to the lessons we can learn from the experience.

Living in the Past

According to writer and lifestyle enthusiast Emily Alvarez, "Your inner critic results from events in your past that you don't want to reoccur." If you've ever felt like a failure or are dealing with other insecurities such as doubt and fear, then you will more than likely feel as though you're on the wrong path. Even though none of us want to struggle, it is going to happen to the best of us.

To move beyond this critic, we need to make peace with the fact that there are going to be times when we fail at things. That's okay as long as we use each of these opportunities to learn. The problem is that the voices inside your head have made you feel that because you've failed once before, you're more than likely to do it again and again, so why should you even bother trying (Alvarez, 2020)?

Celebrate the Wins

Understand this: You simply cannot fail at everything you touch or set your mind to. There have to be areas where you excel, where you are strong, and where you succeed. With our inner critics blaring at us, it's often difficult to recognize those times when we do succeed. It becomes challenging to celebrate each of our victories because the critic within us is trying to make us believe that each of these minor wins is useless, and we should just give up trying.

The scales always seem to be tipped away from success; however, this is unrealistic. We need to look at things logically and reasonably. Are we such a big disappointment to others? Even if you can answer yes to this question, there is still hope for you depending on what you plan to do with the experience you've gained.

Are you putting it to good use to not only educate yourself but possibly those around you? Or are you happy to wallow in self-pity, berating yourself and cursing the situation when it comes to messing up?

Please understand that everyone fails at something sometimes. This is such an important point to reiterate; failure isn't final. It happens to us, but it doesn't have to define who we become.

Whenever those voices in your head start shouting at you that you're going to fail, ignore them. Don't allow any of those fears to hold you back. If you happen to be unsuccessful, there's a valuable lesson to be learned. Whenever this is the case, give it your all. At least at the end of the day, you'll be able to honestly say you gave it everything you've got.

It's understandable that failing at something sucks. Nobody enjoys the experience of defeat. It's worth bearing in mind that by being unsuccessful, other opportunities open up to you. One of these opportunities is growth by learning through your experiences.

Focus on the Positive

It's part of the human condition for us to constantly focus on the negative rather than the positive. That voice in your head that second-guesses every scenario or provides you with a variety of "should haves" instead can certainly cause you to remain stuck in the past.

One of the dangers when it comes to listening to our inner critic all the time is that we lose confidence in ourselves. We run into this inner turmoil where our critics have a go at one another. Our self-confidence takes a complete hammering, and we lose whatever belief we had in our own abilities.

Recognizing our achievements for what they are becomes difficult. We don't believe that we have anything worthwhile to offer the world. Even in the event of many prior successes, we push these aside and focus only on what's currently in front of us (and it's all negative).

This has a knock-on effect when it comes to our sense of achievement. We will need these to keep us motivated and moving in the right direction. Whenever we set goals for ourselves, we need to be able to remain focused on achieving them. Losing focus because we are paying more attention to our inner critic could prevent us from identifying those successes we have accomplished.

According to Jena Pincott from *Psychology Today*, this critic is responsible for a mentality that demands that we either "succeed or suffer." She shares the story of an accomplished young woman who is trying to get into a prestigious law firm. Throughout the interview process, however, she keeps second-guessing herself instead of being confident enough to answer the questions posed to her by the panel. It is her inner critic that keeps her from feeling confident. The unfortunate thing is it is also why this girl has graduated from law school. It has kept her self-disciplined in everything she has achieved in her life to date (Pincott, 2019). Winning marathons. Being the first to go to college in her family. Her inner critic made her push herself further and further to get to where she is today.

This same voice is responsible for the success that many individuals enjoy in life, but as much as it can be a positive influence, it can also turn itself on its head, harming you instead.

Your Inner Critic as a Taskmaster

There's no denying that our inner critic can be demanding. Finding this hard taskmaster has its pros and cons. Some of the pros include being able to push yourself further, knowing what you want to accomplish by the end of the day. Cons, on the other hand, include that you may not necessarily be working to your own set of standards.

One psychologist from California described the inner critic as something extremely challenging to get under control because these voices come across as being from a stern parent (Pincott, 2019).

What we've previously described as "parental voices" eventually become our own, and because we are our own worst taskmaster, a vicious cycle can begin. We start demanding more and more of ourselves. We want things done better, faster, quicker, more accurately, with a sense of perfection—whatever it is, we feel as though we have to raise the bar.

Dealing With Failure

Whenever we fail, the main emotion that's attached is shame. We discover that when we beat ourselves up because we have done something foolish, then whatever can come from the rest of the world can't be that bad. Often, this is because we are harder on ourselves than others. These voices are loud and can be unrelenting when it comes to us feeling competent or worthy of anything. They treat us worse than anyone else ever could.

Some examples of the message that we receive from our inner critic are:

- Shame on you if you don't work hard.
- Shame on you if you're not tougher, smarter, or better.
- Shame on you if you fail, so don't even try (Pincott, 2019).

Remember the young woman interviewing for law firms? She initially saw this harsh critic as something to be proud of. It was something that would spur her on to achieving each of the things that she set out to do in life. However, when it came time to return to the real world after college where things were no longer focused on her getting through college with the best grades possible, she experienced a much harsher reality.

Here, she would be tested by her own belief system in her own abilities. This is where the wheels fell off. All was fine while she was in college doing well, succeeding against her own high standards. However, coming into the real world was more different than she could ever imagine.

This is where we often find ourselves, in a position of fear, unable to move. Fear becomes our new mantra because we know that as long as we are too afraid to do anything, we are in a holding pattern in our lives. While this may make sense to us at the time, it prevents us from celebrating whenever we are successful. Rather than being overjoyed by our accomplishments, we are often only mildly relieved that the situation is over.

This leads us to constantly have high expectations for ourselves that we can never satisfy, leading to anxiety and depression. Can you imagine living under these circumstances? Maybe you are currently in this headspace in your own life right now.

When it comes to the inner critics, they are often so loud that they stifle us from the ability to grow and develop further as an individual. Instead, they keep us stuck in the moment, beating ourselves up over things that could have been. By doing this, we protect ourselves or prepare ourselves for being judged by the rest of the world.

It is this fear that keeps you motivated and moving toward your achievements. However, the inner critic won't allow you to refer to them as achievements just in case this sets you to rest on your laurels, satisfied with yourself and your accomplishments. It prevents you from even acknowledging any form of success whatsoever. The reason for this is to stop you from working through inspiration.

No matter what you do or how hard you try, you won't entirely succeed in getting rid of all of these voices in your head. Studies conducted by the University of Michigan and the University of Berkeley both indicate that there's no point in trying to silence them. No matter how hard you try to get rid of the inner critics in your head, they will keep coming back (Schaffner, 2020).

In the same vein, don't try and overanalyze the various emotions that may have led to the inner critic in the first place. Ethan Cross and Ozlem Ayduk of the above two universities agree that detaching from the critic is one of the best ways to cope with the signals being received. One of the ways to do this is to view the inner voices as though they were a completely different entity.

There are so many different ways that this inner critic is able to prevent us from moving forward. It seems to constantly want to derail us. That's because the message that it puts out there is always negative. The parental nagging that seems to go on forever doesn't have anything positive to say. However, the good news is that we don't always have to listen to what it is saying. We have choices in front of us. As we've discussed in this chapter, we don't have to live in the past. We can celebrate each small victory for exactly what it is without feeling guilty. We can spend our time being productive and focusing on the positive instead of the negative.

In the following chapter, we are going to look at where our thoughts come from and the tremendous power they have over us if we allow them to. By understanding this, we can start taking the first steps toward freeing ourselves from these damaging voices in our heads.

Chapter 3:

The Epicenter of Your

Inner Critic

"We establish most of our self-beliefs during our childhood, but they were based on our limited understanding of the world around us. They are either flawed or have become outdated. We can't take these beliefs at face value anymore."
~ Yong Kang Chan

One of the things I appreciate from the above quotation is that the main time that our inner critic is first introduced to us is when we are children. Things change over time as we get older. We certainly have a much greater capacity to choose our own thoughts and standards, as well as what we believe for ourselves as we grow.

Why, then, do we insist on accepting these inner critics that sit at the heart of who we are? It's often easier. After all, our inner critic has been with us for years since it often stems from experiences during childhood.

Discovering exactly where our inner critic stems from can be a long journey from where we are now back into our childhood days.

We know that our inner critic is controlled by the thoughts we have and the thoughts we allow to take the helm and steer our lives in the direction they want to take us. So, where do these critical thoughts reside? Inside our heads, of course. It's no surprise that we have thousands of thoughts, but trying to pinpoint just one of the thousands running through our heads at any given moment can prove to be even more chaotic than finding our way to our seat at a major baseball event when the stadium is packed to capacity. (Not to mention that you're trying to strategically balance some hot dogs and drinks simultaneously.) We find ourselves in a precarious situation whichever way we choose to slice it.

Among the 50,000 thoughts we're trying to process every day, if the majority of these are negative, critical, and berating, we can often begin to feel overwhelmed. Sifting through these thoughts trying to find that glimmer of hope and that positive thought to keep us moving forward could prove to be more challenging than we initially thought.

Remember that we are constantly processing things walking in and out of our minds like a busy main road. Imagine if each person fighting their way through downtown was an individual, critical thought that you allowed to randomly cross through your mind. Each time they did, however, they made a snide, rude, or judgmental remark. How would that make you feel? Probably not very good.

Whenever your brain is searching for answers to questions that it cannot justify or find, it hits a loop and keeps running these thousands of thoughts over and over and over again until eventually a solution is found. While this happens, you are being hammered by your inner critic constantly.

Most of this self-talk is negative and aimed at breaking down your resolve. Chances are that your brain is currently focused on negative self-talk rather than positive self-soothing. I think that the choice of words being used will ultimately describe the kind of experience you are having. With negative self-talk, you're berating yourself and beating yourself up over virtually nothing. Positive self-talk, on the other hand, will help uplift your mood in every area of your life. The opposite, of course, is to continue feeding your inner critic and allowing it to take control of your beautiful mind.

Because the inner critic is allowed to negatively influence your mind, it is then in a prime position to control what Jennifer Williams, the author of *Goodbye Me Hello Me: Letting go of the past, to embrace your future*, refers to as "our perception of life experiences." She describes how the experiences we have in our lives result in the way that we view the world around us, whether good or bad. Our inner critic plays a role in this by impacting how we experience things and the thoughts we have about them. This would result in a positive or negative life experience (Williams, 2019).

With the number of thoughts going through our heads daily, this could make it increasingly difficult to separate positive thoughts from negative ones. Because we each differ from one another, the self-belief system we potentially inherit from our circumstances would be just as unique.

Consider what your inner mind looks like at this time. Are you constantly filled with negative self-talk? Your thoughts will either motivate you to move forward or keep you in a state where you can keep yourself safe and sane. This is where your emotional regulation system kicks in to either the fight, flight, or freeze mode.

Which of these responses we jump to stems from our upbringing because depending on how we grew up, the way our parents treated us and responded to our needs and situations determined how we react to situations that we are exposed to.

The way we are raised also contributes to our self-esteem. This will help formulate how and what we think of ourselves. These are the thoughts and belief patterns that become how we see ourselves as adults. This forms the backbone of our self-belief system. While we believe that our parents are extremely influential in being the cause of our self-belief system, it's how we perceive each of these encounters with the various role models in our lives that manage to mold these experiences instead.

As children, we are easily molded and shaped by the circumstances and experiences that happen around us. What we identify an experience to be according to our level of understanding could be a catalyst when it comes to developing habits that aren't always in our favor. Our level of understanding as children could be a contributing factor to our limiting belief system.

Some examples may include misinterpretations of different scenarios. For example:

- Your dad happens to be busy with an important project, and you demand his attention. Because of the nature of his work, he simply cannot attend to you immediately. His abrupt response is taken out of context, and as a small child, you believe that he no longer loves you.
- Your mom is in the middle of an urgent phone call, and you want to ask her something. You stand there getting frustrated in front of her until she dismisses you. Once again, your interpretation is one of not being loved. You feel like you are seen as a burden to both parents, having experienced each of these scenarios.
- A teacher happens to be having a bad day and possibly responds to a situation in a classroom

in a volatile way, making you as the student feel small and insignificant.

In these scenarios, there was nowhere that the behavior of the adult indicated hatred or lack of tolerance toward you as a child; however, that's not the way you perceived it to be. It's this perception that we carry with us into the future, and it's this perception that gets in our own way. Can you see how each of these could potentially lead to a form of limiting self-belief that you could carry with you into adulthood?

The way we interpret either dialogue, body language, or a remark may be far removed from the truth; however, it's what we accept to be reality, and because of this, we allow our inner critic to rise.

In each of the above scenarios, the interpretation or experience of the child has been one of anger, frustration, lack of attention, lack of love, and an entire gamut of emotions that are difficult to process. However, it's based on these negative experiences that the inner critic is born. Each scenario resulted in a negative emotion or painful experience. Although we may have experienced these things as a child, they are carried forward into adulthood. While we may have the intention to avoid as much similar pain or discomfort as possible, this is not always how things play out when it comes to internal dialogue.

It's important to accept that your inner critic is what is responsible for your negative self-talk.

It's worthwhile mentioning that it's not just experiences of when we are children that can cause us to form inner critics. Even negative experiences as teenagers or adults can produce an identical effect. Those returning from war or even individuals who have experienced physical abuse and suffer from post-traumatic stress disorder (PTSD) will react differently to certain sounds or situations than those who have not gone through the same type of ordeal.

Understanding the Connection to Thoughts

Rhonda Byrne, the author of *The Secret,* said "your thoughts become things" (Byrne, 2006/2016). We need to understand the connection between what we think and how that can translate into what we do or how we act or react to a given situation. Earlier, we spoke about the reaction that the body has to threatening situations where it will produce the fright, freeze, or flight response. Whenever this happens, the body releases hormones directly related to stress. These hormones are called cortisol.

While you may not be in a life-threatening situation, your brain doesn't realize this because it is acting in line with the thoughts you are having. Because your mind is so powerful, it's important to reduce the number of stressful thoughts and emotions you have. If this process becomes a habit, then your stress functionality or body's inability to deal with constant stress will take its toll on the body, leaving you feeling depleted.

If you insist on taking on stressful emotions constantly, then it will result in creating a barrier to any lasting inner peace and happiness. Stress and negative emotions will reinforce that barrier to happiness. The good news is that you can retrain the way your brain thinks to get your inner critic under control.

Susan Ariel Rainbow Kennedy (SARK), the author of *Creative Companion: How to Free Your Creative Spirit*, describes the attributes of our inner critic as follows:

Inside Critics

The critical voices inside our own heads are far more vicious than we might hear from the outside.

Our "inside critics" have intimate knowledge of us and can zero in on our weakest spots.

You might be told by the critics that you're too fat, too old, too young, not intelligent enough, a quitter, not logical, prone to try too many things…

It's all balderdash!

Some elements of these may be true, and it's completely up to you how they affect you.

Inside critics are just trying to protect you. You can:

Learn to dialogue with them.

Give them new jobs.

Turn them into allies.

You can also dismantle/exterminate them (SARK, 1991).

Your inner critic behaves like a thief in the middle of the night, robbing you of every ounce of self-confidence that you may have had once upon a time. It works with your ego, telling you regularly that whatever you are doing is not good enough. It may whisper in your ears or sound as though it is screaming at you.

The ego could potentially also puff you up. This happens when the ego is stroked to the point where you honestly believe that you can never do anything wrong. This places you in a position where you feel entitled to judge others. This is just as unhealthy as judging yourself. The words that the inner critic uses are as important as if you were speaking them to yourself or your best friend.

Your words are like a thread that forms part of a finely spun spider web. With each word, you could be moving closer and closer to the epicenter where a giant spider may be found. The spider is not something you want to get too close to because it can be something dangerous.

Your thoughts and words can be closely compared to this.

According to psychologist and writer Lynn Newman (2011), an inner critic can potentially have a mantra that it uses to ensure that we become stuck within the web that has been intricately woven into our lives by something that's not real. Here's what this mantra sounds like:

- So what?
- Who cares?
- What's the big deal?
- Why not do things this way?
- What does it matter if I am like this or not?

It doesn't matter who you are or what station in life you come from; you can potentially suffer from an inner critic that's prepared to drown out any normal voice of logic or reason. It also has the nasty habit of making its appearance at the most inappropriate time. The instant you feel that you're second-guessing yourself, then you can be certain that your inner critic has kicked in and is now in full swing.

The Current Social Dynamic

Part of the reason why we can be so hard on ourselves is that we are self-conscious due to the current social dynamic. By this, I'm referring to social media where everyone ensures that they put their best foot forward constantly. All the hype and attention created causes us to become socially awkward individuals as if having a harsh inner critic is not bad enough.

How can you identify whether your current social media habits are fueling your current inner critic rather than allowing it to wash over you like the waves in the ocean? This is easy to figure out. If you insist on checking your profile several times a day to see whether you have received likes, tweets, re-tweets. or been tagged, then you have a problem. Social media has created a society that needs instant gratification to feel complete.

There is more to our social media habits than just remaining in close contact with a circle of friends and family. For others, not receiving instant gratification by sufficient likes or comparing your current lifestyle to the lifestyles of others can cause your inner critic to go on a rampage, letting you know how different your life is compared to others within your social circle. Some of the emotions you could be feeling that will allow you to recognize that they come from your inner critic are things such as shame, anger, jealousy, insecurity, and even regret.

Be aware of all forms of negative emotions because these have originated with your inner critic. There are several examples of these negative emotions mentioned above. This list is by no means exhaustive.

What's Ruminating?

Ruminating is like a constant running commentary that will go on through your mind replaying conversations, decisions, actions, and even events that have happened in your life. It is like looking at a recording of these events where your brain can't put an end to them, so they remain on a constant loop.

This loop is always negative when it comes to ruminating. Another component of this useless activity is that the action, decision, event, or thought has already happened; it is in the past. What happens with thinking about it is that your brain focuses on what might have been, what could have been, or what possibly should have been. It's time to be able to face reality when it comes to ruminating, however, and the truth is that it has already happened, and there's nothing that you can do to make any changes.

Yes, you can change your life moving forward, but that's an entirely different set of necessary skills. First and foremost, you need to move past the ruminating stage of things. The stage where you hold yourself up to the light in such a way that all your faults and flaws are glaringly obvious to everyone you come across. Having the right mindset will allow you to make the changes necessary in your life to bring ruminating to an end. Please understand that there's a big difference between being able to analyze a situation from a healthy perspective and focusing entirely on rumination instead.

Whenever you catch yourself thinking about something that has happened in the past that you know you have no power to change, break the habit by focusing on something entirely different and remove yourself from the environment that's causing you to ruminate in the first place. An important lesson to remember is that when you are ruminating, you cannot be as productive as you possibly could be without focusing entirely on the past. The only thing that the past is good for is remaining there. Don't keep on going back there; you aren't going that way!

"We are what we think. All that we are arises with our thoughts. With our thoughts, we make our world."
~ Buddha

Rumination is always negative. It is always self-defeating and berating. It always makes us that much smaller than we are. There's no benefit to ruminating and listening to the inner critic constantly. We need to be able to be confident enough within ourselves and our own abilities to deal with these inner critics. I mention critics in the plural form because it's rare that an inner critic is limited to only one voice. We spoke about our inner critics being molded and shaped during childhood and what we were exposed to during our earlier years.

Please understand that focusing on the inner critic and the negative voices in our heads for long enough will create the perfect environment for anxiety and depression to begin to form. These are much more serious mental health issues that may require qualified and certified mental health practitioners to work closely with you to deal with self-defeating thoughts and behaviors.

We spoke above that our thoughts become things. Whenever we choose to believe some piece of information that our inner critic is feeding us, we begin to act out according to the way we feel. If our feelings are focused purely on negativity, guess what? That's exactly what you are going to get—a life filled with negativity.

So, what are some of the things that can trigger ruminating thoughts and behavior? These could fall into a multitude of categories throughout our lives and can strike any area without warning. Think about what might go through your mind if you were suddenly faced with divorce or a messy breakup. If you are likely to be listening to your inner critic combined with rumination, then one of the first things you're going to be considering is what a failure you are. You may even wonder what you ever did to deserve being in the relationship in the first place.

Chances are you are going to be looking inward to blame yourself and overanalyze things that you did throughout the relationship rather than pointing fingers at your ex-partner.

If you happen to be particularly stressed out, rumination can occur. This could be a result of the nerves that you're currently experiencing. Rumination is not uncommon if you happen to be facing a life-threatening or life-changing trauma or event. Consider someone who is suddenly diagnosed with terminal cancer. Their entire life is flashing before their eyes, and rumination will be responsible for filling them with remorse or regret for things that they've either done or haven't done with their lives.

Rumination in combination with your inner critic forms quite a dangerous companionship, and it pays to be aware of when your mind decides to go wandering so that it doesn't happen to be in these kinds of directions. You need all of your faculties about you if you plan to beat both your inner critic as well as rumination.

Chapter 4:

Reducing the Negative Effects of Your Inner Critic

"The truth is everything is impermanent. Nothing stays the same. Flowers wither. Our bodies grow old. Even though our thoughts and emotions seem to dissolve over the concept of self, we lose ourselves in the past and don't allow ourselves to just be who we are in the present."
~ Yong Kang Chan

In this chapter, we are going to consider various techniques we can apply in our lives to not become hijacked by the voice(s) in our heads. Before discovering that there are such things as inner critics whose main function seems to be to derail our lives as best they know how and as quickly as possible, the voices we hear may often resemble the voice of a loved one or someone we have respect for. This could be a parental figure, a mentor, manager, teacher, and occasionally even a partner or best friend.

Understanding that all these inner critics are given access to that space in your head by one single entity—yourself—gives it a slightly different perspective. Your inner critic can be controlled only once you know how to control your own thoughts and the behaviors or actions that come from them.

You can begin to transform each of these negative, self-defeating thoughts into positive ones, though. To do so, you must devise a plan of what you want to achieve and by when. Just like any skill, you cannot become a master at something without first learning to walk before learning to run.

Imagine expecting someone to know how to write computer code purely because they happen to have a computer. We can all see that this would be something impossible to do without all the necessary software and skills to boot. That doesn't mean it won't ever be possible. It's just a goal that will need some time to achieve. When plotting out your goals, be sure that they are big enough to frighten you and exciting enough to keep you enthusiastic.

Of course, no problem can be solved without first recognizing that it is a problem. Therefore, when it comes to figuring out this inner critic, one of the first steps is to recognize that you need to do something drastic to rescript the narrative of your life.

Get a Big-Picture Perspective

Sometimes, we struggle to see things that are right in front of us purely because we can't see the full picture. This big-picture thinking can be used to survey those things that need to be altered in our lives. To do this, we need to take several different snapshots of where we are in life and what is surrounding us to see what needs to be improved. Is there anything that immediately strikes you as something you need to work on? If so, that is where you should start.

Imagine for a moment that you are an eagle flying high overhead. You have had plenty of time to survey the landscape that is your life. You can clearly identify those things that are working for you and those things that aren't. If things aren't working out for you, ask yourself what you can do to change that.

Most of the time when you evaluate your situation, you will see that you are juggling your time, effort, and energy when it comes to your harsh inner critic. Are there ways that you can make your life easier? You may also see things that you want to change because they are going to add greater value to your life.

Once you have figured out what you need to do, take the required action and watch your life begin to unfold right before your eyes. Move out of planning mode and into action mode to monitor your progress daily. You should see improvement.

But identifying problem areas isn't always easy to do. You may find that as hard as you try to identify those areas under your inner critic's control, you can't always recognize what is currently out of whack. If you don't know where to look, the problem of your inner critic could remain, and it may be worsened by the frustration you feel.

The good news is there are several ways to quiet your inner critic just by turning the volume down a bit and getting to hear what the other voices inside your head are trying to tell you. One of the best ways is developing mindfulness.

Mindfulness

Think of your mind as one big stage. Thoughts are processed in the same way a director would place each of the main characters in their positions. Dialogue begins to happen that is mainly negative, with the characters berating each other at every opportunity.

Now here's the thing that is so wonderful about your mind. You are able to retrain it and replace each of these characters with others that are more user-friendly. How? With mindfulness.

Mindfulness means being present and living in the current moment rather than batting back and forth between emotional highs and lows because you keep on believing the things your inner critic is choosing to tell you.

One of the things that author Jennifer Williams asserts about mindfulness is that the mind has the potential to create some of the greatest stories imaginable. The big question, though, is whether or not you choose to believe them. You decide whether you should believe them by questioning whether the information that the mind is holding is real or a figment of an overactive imagination.

Remember that what you think about yourself is not true and seldom realistic. Instead of accepting your thoughts at face value, ask yourself whether they are true or not. If the thoughts are valid, then maybe you have something you need to work on. However, if they prove not to be true, then determine what is true and what is the half-truth your inner critic would have you believe.

Think back to that stage and the way the mind has the capacity to direct whichever individual happens to be there at the time. These characters, or thoughts, have the capacity to do and say anything that the mind conjures up regardless of whether or not it is true.

A prime example of this would be when you have messed up something. In this case, this happens to be a legitimate mess, so there's no arguing with your inner critic on that score. Unfortunately, what begins to happen, though, is that each character feels the need to be done in strict compliance and conformity with the mind (Williams, 2019).

This may be the first time you've made a mistake, or maybe it's a mistake that falls in line with your critical expectations. Either way, the verbal abuse, self-sabotage, and self-berating behavior begin. And it is unrelenting. Your inner critic begins holding you responsible for every tiny mistake you have ever made in your life. The sad thing is that because you are human, you will fail at something if not multiple things, and your inner critic will not let them go.

Once you have examined your thoughts, the step that needs to be followed next is known as reframing the situation. In simple terms, this means that you can recognize whenever a negative thought crosses your mind. Remind yourself that in terms of your inner critic, you are being set up for failure. Instead of focusing on the bad or negative scenarios, turn your attention to another 'stage' that happens to be set perfectly for success, where the scenarios are positive and believable.

Reframing is another way of focusing on successes rather than losses. While you may have experienced a loss this time around, you may have been successful before. Pay attention and shift your focus to these times to celebrate your wins rather than your losses.

Remind yourself that no one is perfect, nor will anyone achieve a sense of perfection during this lifetime. You can, however, try to be 1% better every day. This is a simple philosophy of trying to put in a little more effort each day so that you move forward rather than backward (Clear, 2018).

The progress you are likely to experience by doing things a little better each day may seem small, but when it is all added together and compounded, the amount of growth that you will undergo or experience as an individual will be substantial rather than insignificant. This is especially true if you also sit and analyze your current strengths and limitations through self-awareness practices so you know which areas in your life are lacking or in need of growth (Clear, 2018).

Mindfulness practices like what we have talked about take a fair amount of practice to master. It is a daily process that requires constant, consistent intervention and practice. While that may seem daunting at first, it is a powerful tool that can make you feel better about yourself and help you deal with the negative inner critic.

Mindfulness can become a simple routine to implement in your life. Initially, it may not be all that easy to do, especially when you have an overzealous inner critic that's trying to take over the world. The secret lies in being able to close off your mind to as much of the negativity and inner critic rant as you possibly can.

You may not be able to ever stop your inner critic from materializing with its hooks and tentacles as it tries its best to derail your life, but progress can be made, and there are certain benefits that you will experience. You can potentially move from one victory to another, focusing on those things that are positive rather than negative. These changes will certainly influence your personal growth and personal development for the better.

According to Amy Morin, psychotherapist and author of *13 Things Mentally Strong People Don't Do* (2014), there are six specific steps you can take to get your inner critic under control, possibly for good. These six steps are:

1. **Accept yourself for who you are, and balance your personal development.** We have discussed that failure is very much part of life itself. Without failure, none of us would experience growth in any shape or form. You can prepare yourself for these feelings of failure by asking what the worst thing would be if what you are thinking about yourself happened to be true. Surely, this would not mean the end of the world. Yes, it may mean that you need to experience a rather steep learning curve, but apart from this, you have the potential to be able to learn and grow from it.

2. **Avoid pondering over what has happened in the past.** The other word for this, which we've discussed above, is ruminating. Although we have mentioned it, it warrants being mentioned again. Revisiting the past with the intention of making yourself feel bad about things you've done serves no purpose whatsoever. As long as you learn from your mistakes, you should be able to move forward with your life. Ruminating is just pulling your focus away from those things you should be thinking about.

3. **Become aware of your thoughts.** This is a form of self-awareness that is emotional intelligence. You need to pay greater attention to the thoughts you experience at any given moment. This could mean questioning them for validity as mentioned above. It could mean becoming more in tune with the messages you're sending yourself. Remember that just because your inner critic makes a statement or passes judgment doesn't make the belief true.

4. **Evaluate the evidence for accuracy.** If you can truly prove that you are justified in your thinking and the evidence supports your thoughts, then the thought is fine; however, we all know that we are our own worst enemy, and the thoughts we have are often blown way out of proportion. To look for evidence, Morin suggests getting hold of a pen and paper and either writing the thought down or drawing it so that it becomes more visually accurate in your mind. This allows you to determine whether or not you are judging yourself too harshly.

5. **Use accurate statements instead of critical ones.** Reframe your statements by changing negative statements to ones that aren't inflated in any way. If you're thinking something along the lines of "I always mess up when it comes to this," you may know that this is not true

because you have managed to be successful on more than one occasion. You can replace this statement with something along the lines of "I know that I may have missed the mark today, but I will do better tomorrow." Be realistic in whatever you are claiming yourself to be.

6. **Walk in a friend's shoes.** Consider what you would tell a friend to do if you saw them doing some of the things you are currently doing. Imagine that your friend is in a similar situation. What would you tell them or what advice would you give? Chances are if you knew that your friend was going through what you are currently experiencing, you would be loving, supportive, and encouraging. Now, are you willing and ready to take some of your own advice when it comes to this? Consider ways for you to be more understanding toward your inner self.

Inner Chatter

What you say to yourself can move you closer toward achieving your goals or place you in a mode of stasis where you become stuck, unable to move forward or backward. This is possibly one of the most frustrating places to be in, especially when you want to reach goals that you've identified as being important to you.

Each time you run yourself down internally through your inner critic, you are giving some of your power away. This is the power that you need that is going to propel you through life. Without it, you are an empty shell of an individual. While you may reach a degree of potential, it will prevent you from reaching your full potential, and that's not where you want to be.

You want to be able to regulate this inner chatter down to the bare minimum or at least learn how to turn the volume of each of these inner critics down. They can often come across as noisy children that need to be spoken to because they are making too much noise in the background. We all know that some children will be obliging and become aware that their volume is unreasonable, but others will only force themselves to communicate even louder than before, almost doing so in defiance of our needs.

As we deal with our inner critic, we can put ourselves in control of the outcome by being more assertive and dominant whenever we realize that our inner critic is beginning to take control. This takes time and practice, so don't expect to get everything accomplished all in one go. Be realistic about your expectations, and remember that your inner critic has been around for a long time and often knows exactly what buttons to push to set you off.

Chapter 5:

Self-Limiting Beliefs

"You begin to fly when you let go of self-limiting beliefs and allow your mind and aspirations to rise to greater heights."
~ Brian Tracy

Self-limiting beliefs are exactly that. They relate directly back to who we are as individuals and the limitations we decide to put on ourselves. Most self-limiting beliefs are directed inward, so there's no surprise that the language is filled with things like "I am, I can't, I don't, I couldn't." Some examples of typical statements that contain self-limiting beliefs include:

- I can't do that because I don't have enough experience.
- I'm too young.
- I'm too old.
- I'm not qualified to do this.

And this list could easily go on for a number of pages, but you get the idea. You can probably easily come up with a fairly long list of self-limiting beliefs that you say to yourself almost daily. You may not even be aware of the damage you're causing to yourself and how you're also robbing your employer, family, and the world of a valuable resource who could be making someone else's life better were you able to identify that you are doing this and then learn how to stop.

One of the most obvious consequences of limiting self-beliefs is that they place an incredible amount of strain on us in the form of self-induced limitations. If you consider the quotation from Brian Tracy above, you see that you cannot accomplish all the things that you want to achieve if you are holding on to beliefs that you are going to fail.

In this chapter, we are going to take a look at where these limiting beliefs come from and the detrimental effect they can have on our lives. We need to understand how these hold us back and prevent us from achieving some of the goals in our personal and professional lives that we have identified as being important.

As long as you continue to hold on to your limiting beliefs, you won't reach or achieve those things that are important to you.

Something worth mentioning is that for many individuals, they're frustrated at not being able to reach their goals, but they have no clue what's holding them back. This is due to limiting beliefs that are influencing them and their lives, preventing them from achieving everything they want to achieve. They aren't even aware that such beliefs exist, and they have no idea how to get them under control so that they can once again take their place behind the steering wheel of their lives instead of allowing other things to man the wheel.

Understanding Limiting Beliefs

Before we can look at what we can do to bring these under control, it's important for us to get a good idea of exactly what it is that we are looking for. Limiting beliefs are the way we perceive everything around us as well as all the assumptions we make on a daily basis. This could be within our personal lives or as part of our employment.

Beliefs can be dangerous because they influence how we act. With self-limiting beliefs, we think we are incapable of things, so we don't even try. Assumptions, on the other hand, can be even more dangerous, especially if they're directed inwardly toward yourself. These could easily prevent you from accomplishing whatever you set your mind on achieving.

What Are Beliefs?

Our beliefs regarding just about everything are formed from the time we are quite young. Because our early years are formative ones, our brains easily recognize specific patterns and associations in the world around us. Our brains, which are more powerful than any computer, can easily identify and associate certain things with others until these become firmly entrenched in our minds.

We develop belief systems in our lives because they will keep us safe and help us understand the world around us. When we are still little, our parents have a dominant role when it comes to molding and shaping these experiences for us. Some examples of this are rewarding things like good manners and punishing things like bullying or other bad behavior.

We formulate much more complex belief systems drawing from the world around us as we grow older and become exposed to more and more things. Some examples of things that will influence our belief systems are television, movies, books, peers from school, and social media. This list is by no means exhaustive, and I'm sure that once you get to thinking about each of these, the lists will expand.

Core Beliefs

Core beliefs are those formulated while we are still young, and they are so powerful that they have the potential of sticking with us forever. The danger with core beliefs is that some of them are not necessarily true. Instead, they are beliefs that we have decided to focus our attention on. If you come from a home where your parents divorced at a young age and you never had a father figure around, this may result in having trust issues or even relationship issues. A core belief in this type of scenario could be "I'm unlovable because my parents are divorced."

You may have had parental issues where your parents worked long hours to support the family. This could have led to trust issues or feelings where you felt like you were less than worthy of their love and affection because they were never around. Another core belief would be "I am unworthy of love because my parents would rather be spending time at the office than with me."

Some people grow up holding grudges against their parents because they had to hold down multiple jobs to keep the financial wheels of the home turning. While that was necessary, from the perspective of the child or adolescent, the reason the parents were never available was that the child wasn't good enough as a family member to warrant them being around them, especially during those times that mattered.

The child may later come to learn that the reason for the parents not being around was because they were out working to keep a roof over their heads, clothes on their backs, and food in their stomachs. It all stemmed from a deep-rooted love for their children. Despite knowing this, the child may never come to terms with this degree of absenteeism in their lives.

We hang on to our core beliefs as well as what our inner critic is telling us because we desperately need for our thoughts and feelings to be validated. One of the reasons for this is that we don't want to be proven wrong. We need to find every shred of evidence that we can to prove that this was indeed the case.

Take, for example, two sons from the same family. One is about 10 years older than the other. By the time the younger brother is heading into adolescence, the older son has moved out of the house to live on his own. Years later, the two brothers happen to be discussing how they recall their childhood. The older sibling groans and complains that there was never any support from either parent while he was growing up. He remembers school events where he was transported to the event and collected from it thereafter, but he was never supported by the parents in any way.

The younger brother grew up under the same roof with the same parents who had the same philosophy on life and the same exacting standards of raising their children. This son remembers his childhood as slightly different. He recalls being supported by the parents in anything and everything he wanted to do. His parents were often required to work during times when there were school sports or other activities taking place, but he understood this.

The first child held a grudge against his parents his entire life. Now, as an adult, he still cannot bring himself to accept that the parents acted in the same way when it came to raising each of their children. In some ways, his life turned out to be a direct reflection of how he perceived his own parents. With his children, he was also absent during those times when he was needed most. If you had to ask him today, however, he would tell you that he was a wonderful parent.

Discovering that our belief system is formed at a young age can be quite frightening. Many of these beliefs that molded and shaped our lives were things we learned when we were in kindergarten. As a result, we need to be sensible about which of these beliefs we are going to hold on to.

An example of this would be learning that it's not right to break another child's crayons. As an adult, we don't necessarily work with crayons. But the basic philosophy of having learned to respect the property of those around us is one we carry through into adulthood. Make sense?

How you were reared as a child will carry through and feed your belief system as an adult. Any form of neglect or abuse could be extremely harmful and impact you into adulthood. You may feel that because this is the way that you were treated as a child, it's the only way for you to get what you want or need from those around you as an adult.

Your home environment may have been as close to perfect as you could have wanted it to be, yet there could still be toxic or limiting self-beliefs passed on to you. Things like having your parents step in and fight every one of your battles for you. This could leave you feeling weak or incapable of being self-sufficient or defending yourself when situations call for it. You may be an emotional wreck when having to face confrontation head-on. You will simply not be prepared for it emotionally or mentally. Parents are certainly doing their children a disservice by not allowing them to fight their own battles.

An important thing to remember about beliefs, though, is that they are not necessarily correct. The problem is that despite beliefs not always being true, they still determine how we choose to act or react to situations in our lives.

Limiting self-beliefs can hold us back from pursuing our dreams; they can prevent us from applying for that promotion we've always wanted. They can stop us from pursuing the man or woman we love all because we don't feel worthy enough.

When we choose to limit ourselves with where we could go or what we could or should believe, we prevent ourselves from gaining traction in our lives and being able to move in the direction of our goals. Self-limiting beliefs prevent us from reaching our goals.

In the Workplace

We've discussed where self-limiting beliefs come from and how we can carry them into adulthood with us.

Now, let's take a deeper look at how these can impact us and prevent us from achieving our goals in the workplace.

What we believe will lead to how we behave, act, and react in a given situation. Unfortunately, it also can sometimes hold us back and prevent us from doing something.

In the section above, we mentioned that feeling unworthy or inexperienced can prevent us from applying for that promotion at work. This is just a simple example of how we can become frozen in the moment or stuck rather than moving toward our dreams of success, especially in the workplace.

Let's take a closer look at some typical excuses that our limiting belief system can be responsible for.

I don't have the money. Yes, this can often be a real situation that holds people back from moving toward their goals. It is not an impossibility though. There are several things that you can do to make it possible to do what you want. This could range from seed funding to applying for short-term finance with a bank to start up a business.

I lack the qualification or experience for this position. The truth is that we all have to start somewhere. You may not have a qualification, but you may have the experience and expertise that are required to do the job at hand. Alternately, you may have the piece of paper with all the technical know-how and you now need someone to guide you with the practical hands-on experience.

In this scenario, the ideal solution to both problems could lie in finding a suitable mentor, someone who has what you need. If you need the qualification and need to hone some of your skills so they are slightly more professional, speak to a mentor about this. If you need someone to mentor you and show you the practical ropes of the business, try and find someone who has a lot of practical experience, and get them to share their knowledge with you. Either way, there is a practical solution to this perceived problem.

I have no motivation. We all hit brick walls from time to time when it comes to keeping ourselves motivated. Looking at solopreneurs and entrepreneurs, it's often difficult to imagine that they ever have a down day because they constantly look and sound as though they are fully charged and motivated 100% of the time. This is not always true. What they have learned to do, however, is to recognize when their motivation levels are beginning to hit a slump, and they then figure out how to deal with it at the time.

One of the characteristics that all highly motivated individuals have is that they are constantly filling their minds and bodies with only the best of everything. Mentally, they are stimulated by material that is positive, motivational, and uplifting. They watch their health and their diet. In general, they take care of each area of themselves mentally, physically, emotionally, and spiritually.

I don't have time. We often complain that we simply do not have enough time available for us to do what is required of us. Sure, demands on our time may be high on the list of priorities; however, we each have the same number of hours, minutes, and seconds in a day. It's what we choose to do with this allotted time that is important.

You will find that most successful individuals have time specifically carved out for themselves, so they manage to get the most out of every moment available to them. And yes, there will always be curveballs thrown, and things that we planned may need to be moved and shifted around to accommodate whatever emergency has been thrown our way. Those who know how to manage their time effectively can take this in stride. Believe me, just as everyone had to start at the beginning of their careers learning as they went along, time management is similar to this.

My age is against me. Let's just call this as it is! Anyone who uses their age as an excuse is doing exactly that—making an excuse. The truth is that you can accomplish whatever it is that you want to accomplish no matter your age. Just turn on the news, and you will see child entrepreneurs and seniors in their 80s who are still gaining qualifications and running their own businesses. The bottom line is if you are dedicated to a specific cause, you will find a way to accomplish whatever it is you need to achieve.

There are others better suited to this position than me. While this may definitely be true, there may be specific gifts and abilities that you bring to a particular position that the other individual may not have. Don't be so quick to discredit those qualities that you possess and how they may contribute toward the overall objectives of a role within an organization.

Once again, this is not an exhaustive list of reasons or excuses that we use as self-limiting beliefs to hold ourselves back or to justify our actions or lack thereof.

We tend to want to hold ourselves to a much higher standard than those around us do. Now, I'm not saying that it's a bad thing to have certain standards that you'd like to aspire to. This is always a positive thing. What isn't acceptable is when you constantly put yourself down because you simply cannot recognize any of the talents or abilities that you have. You are more content to sit waiting in the wings than taking center stage when it comes to playing a leading role in your own life.

If you are waiting until you can do something perfectly every time before you even attempt taking on additional responsibilities in your life, then you are going to be waiting a long time. Nobody is ever able to do everything perfectly all the time; this is an absolute impossibility. If this is the way that you are approaching your life personally and in business, I have two words for you–STOP IT!

Chapter 6:

How to Overcome Limiting Beliefs

"There is one grand lie—that we are limited. The only limits we have are the limits we believe."
~ Wayne Dyer

I want to tell you a story about a baby elephant. While I am not entirely sure where this story originated, I know that what happens in the story is practiced by various circuses as well as zoos and places that have elephants.

As a baby, the elephant is chained to a stake that has been hammered into the ground. It usually has one of its legs chained to the stake using a chain or thick rope that a baby elephant could never free itself from.

As much as the baby elephant attempts to free itself, nothing works, and eventually, the elephant accepts that its fate is to remain fastened to the post. By the time the elephant is fully grown, it no longer attempts to free itself, even though it easily could since it is so big and strong. The reason the elephant no longer attempts to free itself is that it has been conditioned to remain there. It has a belief system that it cannot free itself, so it no longer even tries.

But what does an elephant have to do with us? Like the elephant, we grow accustomed to our self-limiting beliefs, and eventually, we no longer try to challenge them. We believe that they are facts, so we simply accept them.

Unfortunately, these limiting beliefs bleed into how others treat us as well. If we plan on being extra hard on ourselves or demanding that everything we do is perfect, we shouldn't be too surprised when those around us treat us the same way.

So, are you just stuck living with these limiting beliefs forever? Thankfully, there are several ways that you can try and overcome the limiting beliefs that you are insisting on holding on to. And while it may be difficult to overcome a limiting belief, it's not impossible. It takes dedication and effort.

Before we look at some suggestions, let's briefly consider positive and negative beliefs and how they impact us.

Road Signs

Beliefs can either be positive or negative. When beliefs are positive, you can find yourself moving ahead in life at a reasonable speed. On the other hand, negative belief systems will result in you veering off course suddenly. You may find yourself hitting the brakes for no reason whatsoever.

It could be compared to trying to find an obscure location without your GPS. You are likely to make a whole lot of wrong turns before you find the right location, if you manage to find your destination at all.

If you don't know where it is that you are wanting, how can you possibly know which destination you need to be moving toward?

Solutions to Limiting Beliefs

As I said above, you can challenge these negative limiting beliefs and free yourself from them. To start, get creative with other beliefs.

How do you do this? The first thing would be to get to the heart of what your limiting belief is. Once you get there, try and challenge that belief by suggesting something as an alternative to that belief system. What do I mean by this? Here's a simple example. You currently believe that you are too old to begin a new career or go out on your own as a solopreneur. Challenge this belief by doing a bit of a deep dive on the internet. Google will prove just how many successful entrepreneurs broke into the market well into their 50s with some even entering the market for the first time in their 70s and 80s.

Okay, so now that we've got that one out of the way, let's check the whole 'age' thing off the list. When it comes to finding other creative solutions, refer back to some of the limiting beliefs that we listed in the previous chapter, and try to come up with a creative solution that could potentially solve the problem.

Once you've managed to think of creative alternatives to your beliefs, test them out. Here, you are going to try and validate what you have identified as a creative concept or solution to your problem. To test it against your limiting belief, search for evidence of others who have managed to overcome the same thing. How did they manage to do this? Is there something in what they did that you could also possibly recreate? Can you copy their winning formula to help you in your own limiting belief?

This may seem daunting, but consider the following story. Makeup mogul Mary Kay Ash was already in her 50s when she launched her famous brand. What was her reason for starting a multi-level marketing company for cosmetics at that age? Well, she had worked in the multi-level marketing industry for years and been successful at what she did. Her motivation to move out on her own was the fact that she was passed over time and time again for senior promotions within the business, often having to train junior staff members for management roles.

Tired of empty promises within a male-dominated industry, she decided to go against the grain of "politically correct business" in Texas at the time. She borrowed $5,000 for cosmetic raw materials and found herself a reliable chemist who was experienced in working with chemicals and turning them into cosmetic products. The result–the start of the Mary Kay beauty line of cosmetics, one of the most successful multi-level marketing enterprises in the US at the moment. As they say in the classics, the rest is history.

Her company grew because she refused to give in to the limiting beliefs that said as a woman, she would or should never be promoted into a management role within a business. We are so grateful that she never gave up on her vision and her dream.

But what happens if the voice in your head that's telling you that you're too fat, too ugly, not smart enough, or too inexperienced is all that you continue hearing? It's gotten to the point that you are almost ruminating on these things daily. How do you stop that? Throw in this question: What if you are wrong?

Sometimes, we need to stop ourselves and consider the worst-case scenario. Maybe we are wrong. If we are wrong, how is this going to change the outcome for us?

What could we be doing in the interim to set ourselves up for success rather than self-limiting defeat?

Say you have been imagining that you are not good enough, attractive enough, or smart enough. Challenge those beliefs. Since there's a lot for you to be asking yourself in this section, grab your journal or a piece of paper to help. Begin asking some of these questions, no matter how desperately uncomfortable they may be.

Also consider this question: What is the payoff for this belief? This is possibly one of the most challenging questions to ask yourself. However, when you keep on beating yourself over your head and being self-destructive in the process of implementing your limiting beliefs, then there comes a time when you need to ask yourself what the payoff is for hanging on. What are you getting out of it?

This could be something as simple as getting attention from those around you. You'd be amazed by how many people need to have those egos of theirs stroked just to make them feel better about themselves.

Occasionally, it's because we are happy to play the victim card. We carry our hearts on our sleeves, and we want others to pay attention to us. This is not to say that what we are doing is correct. It's the opposite. Anyone pandering using the victim card needs to take a serious look at themselves and where they are currently situated and want to go.

This is yet another pointer where you will benefit from making use of your journal during some quiet time. Use some of your meditation time to find the answers to these questions because they require some deep and serious introspection.

None of these beliefs should be taken purely at face value. You must be prepared to physically do the work to break free from the mold and chains of some of these limiting belief systems. Once you start analyzing more closely, you will discover that there is a lot more work to overcoming limiting belief systems than just acknowledging that they are there.

It is going to take serious introspection and implementing positive habits that can reinforce positive beliefs to replace each of the limiting beliefs that you have. Remember when I mentioned right at the beginning of the last chapter that limiting beliefs all start with personal words like "I am, I can't, I shouldn't"? Break the mold when it comes to these negative self-directed habits first.

Own Your Limiting Beliefs

One of the ways of getting past your limiting beliefs is by choosing to own them, much like we spoke of responsibility and accountability in the previous chapter. When it comes to limiting beliefs, these can get personal because they are mostly directed at us.

As mentioned above, some of the limiting beliefs were adopted at a young age. The longer we've been hanging on to these limiting beliefs, the more challenging it is for us to break free from them. Only when we accept and own our limiting beliefs can we begin to do something about them.

To do that, understand that it is you and you alone that is holding yourself back. You need to be prepared to accept responsibility for your beliefs and your actions.

Monitor Your Internal Dialogue

Another method of overcoming these limiting self-beliefs is by becoming aware of our internal dialogue. This is what we say to ourselves. Below are some examples of common traps we fall into when talking to ourselves.

Thinking in Black and White: Unable to find the middle road in any situation. In other words, if something wasn't an absolute success, then it has to be a complete failure. We all know that this is never the case.

Predicting Disasters: Permanently anticipating that the worst is going to happen. Anticipating disaster at every turn.

Disregarding Positives: If someone pays you a compliment, you ignore it and focus on something negative instead, or you turn the positive compliment into something that's negative.

Emotional Analysis: Analyzing everything by making use of emotions and feelings to determine whether something is true or not. An example of this would be that you think you have large feet, which automatically translates into a fact–your feet are large. This may not necessarily be true. It is purely how you happen to be feeling about a part of your body.

Fortune-Telling: Predicting the outcome of something rather than attempting it for yourself because you are convinced that you're going to fail.

Characterizing: Judging others and being convinced that you are being set up for failure. The moment that someone treats you slightly differently, you imagine the worst.

Being Demanding: A way of thinking where you keep putting your emotions down. Examples of this would include "could have, would have, should have, didn't" styles of thinking and how they can potentially hold you back.

Psychological Filtering: Being permanently focused on the negative rather than the positive. Taking the negative to the next level.

Self-Labeling: Being prejudiced toward yourself. This could include applying names and labels to yourself that aren't accurate. Despite their inaccuracy, you chose to apply derogatory terms to yourself anyway.

Making Assumptions: Assuming responsibility for things that go wrong when they are out of your control. Despite the fact that you aren't responsible in any shape or form, you still assume responsibility.

One way to deal with this internal dialogue that we all have is identifying what it's trying to say to us. Whenever our internal dialogue is negative, chances are that it's going to lead to us feeling bad about ourselves, and we need to do something to break the vicious cycle that it can become.

A big part of solving any negative dialogue is by changing your mindset to something that is more positive. The simple act of putting a smile on your face can immediately turn what has potentially been a negative mood into something that's more positive and upbeat.

Shift Your Mindset

Your mindset is the way you think or feel about certain things. Nothing about limiting beliefs is positive. As a matter of fact, the first part of the phrase clearly states that it's limiting, which indicates that you will only be able to go so far with it. There are barriers, and one of these definitely happens to be preventing happiness. So, how do you go about creating a shift in your mindset?

One of the first things that should be considered is that this is completely your decision. Often, you become frustrated with yourself because you are battling to complete a task or you're not even sure why you decided to pursue the task to begin with. Whenever limiting beliefs crawl in during a project or task, you immediately lose focus and start questioning your own ability to do whatever you originally set your mind to. You find it challenging to assume responsibility and accountability for these feelings or emotions.

Having core values will help you sort through loads of emotions and make some of those difficult decisions. This can help you remain anchored in the present moment rather than getting carried away with things that are unimportant.

Limiting beliefs are unreliable at best. It doesn't matter how much you want for something to be true, if they aren't true, then they simply aren't, and there's nothing you can do about it. This is what keeps people in relationships they don't necessarily want to be in. It keeps people in the same type of job for longer than they should be. Limiting beliefs can stop people from living the life of their dreams, mainly because they don't believe that they deserve to be happy. Individuals stuck in this belief system hold themselves back from pursuing their dreams.

By increasing your self-awareness, you can begin to focus on those things that you are unaware of. This is a form of emotional intelligence that can stand you in good stead when it comes to making decisions and choices that are in your best interests. It helps you to figure out your emotions. Emotional intelligence can help you when it comes to figuring yourself out internally.

Your limiting beliefs are keeping you from living your best life. It's important to understand that beliefs are not necessarily true. They are exactly that, a belief system.

Through self-awareness, you can be aware of unwelcome emotions that accompany these beliefs or may lead to them. These may not always be immediately apparent, which is why you need to be especially cognizant that they may be around.

Watch for patterns. If you are able to focus sufficiently, you may be able to spot them in places. Keep accurate notes so that you are aware when they begin to occur on a regular basis. If you can begin to recognize patterns and possible triggers that set these limiting beliefs off, then you may be able to get them under control.

Don't attempt to do things that you aren't capable of. Remember what your limitations are without being too hard on yourself.

If you catch yourself coming across a limiting belief, then try and replace it with a belief that is empowering instead. Find something that you are good at, and use this to remind yourself of each of the small victories. It's important to be able to celebrate each victory. They are important for your personal progress no matter how small and insignificant they may seem to you.

Redirect your belief system inward. It's important to be able to identify each of your abilities and make use of these. Whenever you find yourself battling some of your self-limiting demons, remember what strengths you have, and don't forget to tap into each of these.

Figure out where the volume control button is when it comes to your limiting beliefs. You need your limiting beliefs to be able to take a back seat or become so silent and in the distance that an empowering belief system replaces them.

Also, consider a different result than one that is linked to your limiting belief. Imagine that this result is possible regardless of your current situation. Use your imagination to the best of your ability. Make use of all of your senses until you can virtually feel and taste this becoming your reality. Consider what it would be like to become the person you truly want to become. Has the image become crystal clear yet? If not, sharpen it. If so, this is the image that you need to be holding in your brain to ensure that this is believable. Remember that if you can see it, you can achieve it.

Consider various opportunities where you would be able to make use of each of your newly honed talents. And remember to celebrate your wins and be proud of who you are becoming.

Limiting beliefs only serve one purpose, and that's to derail you when it comes to meeting your goals and finding happiness. Aim to shift your mindset away from being focused on those limiting beliefs. Increase your self-confidence to the point where it assists you in your fight against limiting beliefs. Focus on developing beliefs that are empowering and will get you to where you want to be. Beliefs, once mastered, can become extremely powerful, and learning how to overcome your limiting beliefs can lead you to a happy, successful, and fulfilled life.

Chapter 7:

Facing Fear

"Each of us must confront our own fears, and must come face to face with them. How we handle our fears will determine where we go with the rest of our lives. To experience adventure or to be limited by the fear of it."
~ Judy Blume

One of the biggest barriers or obstacles to success is fear. Because of this, there are times when we don't even try. We prefer to remain safe and sound in our comfort zones because that way, we don't need to overextend ourselves or try new things. We don't need to overcome any fears of failure because we are just not going to do it.

Can you see how having fears and phobias can easily prevent us from moving forward? While we may often feel that we are unique and have a different set of fears than those around us, in truth, everyone is afraid of something. It's the way that we deal with each of these fears that will either stand us in good stead and keep us moving forward or hold us back.

According to Adam Smith, the author of *Bravest You: 5 Steps to fight your biggest fears, find your passion and unlock your extraordinary life,*

> At some point – present or past – fear has torn us all away from some significant accomplishment or victory. Fear will often keep us running away from things, instead of running toward the goals that we want to achieve.

Obstacles to Success

Smith describes a number of things that we fear that are obstacles to us achieving what we want. Pay attention to the following list, and notice if any of them apply to you.

Being Judged: We've all been there when we've had to read or present something to a class full of peers at school and things suddenly went awry. Maybe the class started laughing or giggling, and you made a decision then and there that they were judging you. You didn't like the feeling of being made to feel small and insignificant. As a result, you decided you would never stand up in front of a crowd again. This has hampered your progress within your career as you love your job, but there are certain tasks that need you to be able to present information to others. Because of one singular event when you were a child, you simply cannot bring yourself to do it.

Change: This could be anything from changing habits to become a better person, physical changes such as in a relationship status, changing jobs, or moving homes. Psychologically, experiencing change is on the same kind of scale as experiencing the loss of a loved one. Be kind to yourself while you are in the midst of change. You want to come out on the other end as a better person rather than someone who is a nervous and emotional wreck.

Failure: This is probably the biggest and worst type of fear you could ever experience. I think it's because it attacks you on so many different levels. Initially, you have failed at a goal that's important to you. But you may also have failed at doing something relatively straightforward that you feel should be easy. Or you may have failed someone close to you such as a parent, partner, friend, employer, or spouse. Fear of failure holds most of us back and prevents us from even trying. Chances are that we have been in a similar position before and failed. That's all we need to convince ourselves to remain on the outside looking in versus active participation.

Getting Hurt: This is another reason why we don't put everything out there, especially when it comes to relationships or our feelings. We are too afraid of getting hurt, and the pain of remaining single is definitely less than the pain of being with someone and then losing them.

Inadequacy: There's nothing quite like discovering that we don't have all the necessary skills or talents required to complete an assignment or task. There are a couple of ways you can go about dealing with this. The first is to admit that you do not have enough skills and are prepared to get out there and make things happen for yourself by learning how to do so. The second is to try anyway and learn from your mistakes as you go. Either way, this is bound to be a learning experience for you and one where you will come out having learned either a new skill or something about yourself.

Losing Control: This can be a major problem for many of us where we are unable to keep our emotions under control. It can result in us lashing out or trying to get attention that we believe we deserve (which is not always true). By being able to keep things under control is something we need to constantly work at.

Missing Out: There is a catchphrase that is currently popular, fear of missing out or FOMO. This is where an individual believes that other people are having fun without them, so they feel the need to always be connected and know what others are doing. This should be handled with care because you don't want to alienate individuals, but you also need to have certain standards met when trying to face this fear head-on.

Rejection: We have all experienced rejection at some time or another, and quite frankly, it sucks. While you don't want to be rejected continuously, rejection often provides us with opportunities where we can learn and grow even more rather than merely going through the motions of trying to pick up the pieces. Rejection can come in many different forms, and it is often more than what we believe it to be. Rejection can be experienced when applying for a new position or promotion, in a relationship, or even the initial advance when trying to meet someone and talking to them. The big thing about rejection is that we have all been there, and if you haven't experienced rejection just yet, it is one thing that will rear its nasty head.

Something Bad Happening: This is often a feeling that begins in the pit of your stomach, or you may find that your heart is suddenly in your throat. It seems like the universe is trying to warn you that there is trouble, and you need to be super vigilant. Some call this intuition or a sixth sense, and the reality is that we all have it. This is that nagging voice in your head trying to warn you that there's either a curveball or danger ahead. This is not the typical voice that you hear in your mind. Instead, this one comes through with crystal clarity and usually has all the necessary tools to be able to take this feeling on.

Uncertainty: Sometimes, the two of these could go hand in hand. When you have a sensation that something's about to go wrong, there's usually a sense of uncertainty that accompanies it. Remember that just because this is the way that you happen to be feeling doesn't mean that it is correct. It simply indicates that you have the wisdom and fortitude to recognize that there may be something that you don't understand coming up.

Success: Would you believe that there are even people out there who are afraid of what would happen should they suddenly become successful? These individuals have been living in doubt and desperation for such a long time that they simply cannot even begin to imagine what the achievement of their goals and success may both look and feel like to them (Smith, 2017). In the chapter that follows, we will dive a little deeper into ways to overcome some of these fears, providing you with workable solutions.

The Psychological Connection

Psychologists are trying to discover the relationship between fear and anxiety. If you consider someone who is on the verge of paranoia (a degree of fear), this is heightened anxiety. While this debate is ongoing, they still haven't found where these two interact with each other just yet.

One of the main things that fear does is affect the way you use your emotions. Once it has taken over your emotions, your decision-making abilities tend to go out the window.

Another thing that fearful people are afraid of is putting themselves out there to take a chance or to risk something. Once again, this is a fear of failure that places them in this state of paralysis where they feel that they're stuck. They can't go forward, and they don't want to go backward either.

Fearful people suffer from being way more pessimistic than optimistic. They are constantly viewing the world as though there's something that's about to go wrong rather than considering all the things that could go right. All that this does is prevent them from living their best life possible because they are so certain that everything they touch is going to be a failure. Because of this, they choose to do nothing instead. Does this sound like you?

We all understand that for us to survive, we need to be able to identify certain levels of fear. It needs to become part of who we are; otherwise, our fight-flight-freeze cortisol-filled moments cannot occur. The point is that this level of fear is there to protect us physically in real life or death situations. We are meant to be experiencing these feelings because this is what will end up keeping us alive.

For us to become successful, we need to be able to push past our fears. We know that there will always be things that we need to be afraid of. But rather than giving in to our fears, we need to be able to harness them and get through them. This will take us one step closer to being able to reach our goals.

But what do you fear? When you analyze your fears, you can probably divide them up into physical fears, psychological fears, and perceived fears.

Physical fears could include things such as public speaking or standing in front of a group of board members presenting a report. Psychological fears, on the other hand, are those fears that play on the mind. They are also not necessarily true, but they make us feel as though we are paralyzed in the moment. This could be things such as being afraid of success for various reasons that seem to make sense to us at the time; however, upon closer inspection, they have no merit whatsoever.

Many individuals experience what can best be described as perceived fears. Some of these present themselves in the form of phobias—fear of heights, being confined in small spaces, spiders, and the list can potentially go on. Even these perceived fears have a special place when it comes to working through our emotions. We cannot begin to process any of our feelings unless we can identify where they come from.

Fear is something that is real and can become overpowering. It can take control of the direction your life is heading in unless you can get it under control. It is possible to redirect your fears and replace what are currently damaging scenarios with healthier options.

We are going to look at solutions to our fears throughout the next chapter, but it is worth mentioning here that there is hope for each of us. Our fears, even those that are the most stifling and crippling, serve a purpose in our lives despite the way we may feel about them right now.

We need to be aware of several things when it comes to fears. First, they are all in our minds. Second, unless we are facing life-threatening danger, we feed our fears. We give them the power that they need to take control over our lives and prevent us from moving forward.

Being in a constant or continual fearsome state will prevent you from being able to live your best life. It robs you of opportunities and keeps you in that stagnating, holding pattern that we spoke about earlier. You don't want to find yourself permanently in this condition as it's not conducive to a constructive and positive life.

We each deserve to live a life that's free of fear. We deserve to know what it feels like to be able to take advantage of all the good things that life has to offer us.

Please understand that one of the things that we cannot do when it comes to fear is to ignore it. This would be not only silly, but it would also add to the current level of fear and uncertainty we are already experiencing.

Above, I mentioned that you may have the feeling that "something's about to go wrong." This is linked to a type of fear that is intuitive. We make use of our intuition to sense when we are in real danger. This is one of the reasons why we should never disregard sensations that we have that may be screaming out at us that we are heading into dangerous territory.

The difference between the two is being able to determine what type of fear you are experiencing and whether it has a valid place in your life. This is especially true when it comes to being intuitive about things that could potentially be on the horizon. Accept the different types and levels of fear that you experience every day, and try and separate them into different groups. This will help you as you work to try to make each of them manageable.

We are going to discuss ways to overcome each of these fears in the next chapter; for now, please accept that there is hope for a life free of all unnecessary fear.

How Fear Can Hinder Us

While we've discussed why we need to have fear as part of our primal response to keep us alive, there are a whole lot of other things that fear is really good at that are not necessarily great for us in the long run. These include:

Excuses: Our fears can help us become masters at making excuses for why we can or can't do certain things. It gives us reasons to keep us stagnant. While some of these excuses may occasionally be valid, in most circumstances, they are creating stumbling blocks and barriers to reaching those goals that we have set for ourselves.

Mental Blocks: Fear can feed into our mental blocks, preventing us from being able to see a way past them. Whenever we hit a mental block, we need to have the foresight and tenacity to realize that there are several ways that these can be dealt with. We can either go over, under, around, or directly through them. A mental barrier is exactly that. Something that is stuck in our minds, and there's nothing to say that whatever we have been thinking about these barriers is true.

Goals and Dreams: Fear will prevent us from reaching those goals and dreams that are especially important to us. Remember that we mentioned fear of failure and fear of success above. Each of these scenarios can be applied when it comes to achieving our goals and dreams. Think about ways that you can overcome both of these rather than having these two obstacles stymie you in one place for an indefinite amount of time.

Limitations: The limitations that fear places on each of us can be situational and change from one individual to the next. However, when we focus so intently on our limitations rather than our strengths, we automatically derail our intentions to move toward our goals. We all have limitations, and they are necessary for us to grow and develop; however, when we choose to allow our limitations to rule our lives without attempting to do something about them, then we are headed down a pretty slippery slope.

Subconscious: This is one of the most important areas when it comes to fear because this is where it all starts. The fear that we become most accustomed to begins in our subconscious until we give it the attention it screams for. Only then can these fears move from our subconscious to our conscious minds. This is where they begin to overpower us, derail us, and draw our focus and attention away from our actual goals and just about everything in between.

When our fears are at the subconscious level, it is difficult for us to identify exactly where the fear is coming from. To do that, we need to be able to move these fears into our conscious realm. However, this is where they gain their power to physically influence the things we do and say, how we act or react to certain situations, as well as take hold of our emotions. This is probably one of the most crucial elements of working through our fears.

Mockery: Here's another one of the fears that can make us feel small and insignificant. This could also be closely linked to some of the first fears that we discussed at the beginning of this chapter. Let's face it, none of us want to be the butt of people's jokes or have individuals pointing and laughing at us. This is what mockery, scorn, and ridicule are all about. Even thinking about it is enough to bring a knot to the pit of your stomach. Do your best not to worry about the noise that others make in response to your efforts. Unless they are someone important in your life, what they think of you and the way they view you should have no bearing on the situation whatsoever.

There have been many different examples of fear that have been given to you as part of this chapter, and you can see how each of these has the potential to make your life completely miserable. The most important thing, though, is to not allow them to get the better of you. How? There are a number of ways of dealing with each of these fears, and we will go through them in greater detail in the following chapter.

Let's dive in and see how you can overcome fear and get to live a much better life than you are currently living. Get ready to accomplish the goals that you have identified for yourself and stay in control of situations rather than allowing them to control you.

Chapter 8:

Overcoming Fear

"I learned that courage was not the absence of fear, but the triumph over it. The brave man is not he who does not feel afraid, but he who conquers that fear."
~ *Nelson Mandela*

Throughout chapter 7, we discussed a plethora of factors that are responsible for causing us to become fearful, afraid, anxious, and, at times, even depressed. These can lead to us procrastinating because rather than tackling our fears head-on, we prefer to skirt around them hoping they'll go away on their own because we're afraid of them.

Only when they don't will we finally venture out to see how many of our challenging fears we can take on with a degree of safety. We don't want to be hurt, which we can often see coming along with many of the challenging situations that life throws our way, and fear is what's preventing us from moving forward and achieving those worthwhile goals in life.

To be successful at overcoming the negative thoughts and fears that we have, we need to first recognize where our fear comes from. You may assume that fear comes from an external source, but that's not always the case.

Recognize Where Fear Originates

Fear is simply deep within us. You and I are responsible for creating our own fear and the specific degree of fear within ourselves. I know that this sounds crazy, but stop and think about this for a second. We imagine negative situations, picture the worst-case scenarios, tell ourselves we will fail—all of these lead to internal fears that control our lives.

This is common knowledge among personal trainers and life coaches alike, which is why if you work with any of them, they will push you to overcome your fears so that you can achieve the success you want. Perhaps Jack Canfield, a life coach, sums it up best with this saying: "Everything you've ever wanted is on the other side of fear."

Of course, there are other reasons for us being afraid when it comes to taking action. Some of these we discussed in chapter 7, but I would like to look at them here from the perspective of being able to control them or try and repair any permanent psychological damage that they may have done.

The biggest fear that we probably hold on to quite tightly is the fear of rejection from others. Whether this is in a work-based environment or in our personal lives, we don't want to let down those who are counting on us. So, in this situation, we decide that the next best thing to do is to simply do nothing. That way nobody can be disappointed with our attempt at doing something. Instead, they get to be disappointed for a whole lot of other reasons.

This fear of rejection can bring a lot of other familiar emotions with it. When I say familiar emotions, I'm not talking about pleasant ones, but they are known to us, and this is why we prefer to not try rather than give things a go when we know they are in our best interests.

You may have been disappointed before or even singled out and made an example of. Neither of these scenarios is comfortable, but to get to the other side of fear, there comes a time when you need to let these things go.

People often spend an inordinate amount of time trying to figure out exactly where their fear is rooted or where it originates in the first place. Here's the kicker: Our fears all stem from ourselves. They are self-inflicted. Just like we are responsible for placing limiting beliefs on ourselves, we are also responsible for setting ourselves up for failure by fearing any form of failure. It doesn't matter which way you slice it, the word 'fear' itself is never going to instill confidence within you to go out of your way and try to do something better, perform better, or strive for higher things. This can only begin to occur if and when you manage to get your fear under control.

Fear is something that we have imagined for ourselves, and it includes conjuring up numerous scenarios that we continue to dwell on. Is this to say that what we currently believe in is likely to come true? Chances are, more often than not, that what you fear won't come true because it is just a figment of your imagination after all.

We manage to place ourselves in a position where we are paralyzed by fear, though, because we allow our imaginations to run wild. Since we worry about the unknown future, we try to predict exactly what the future has in store for us, and most of the time, we assume that it's nothing good, which prevents us from moving forward.

All of this overthinking is hazardous for our health. We are in an environment where there's no telling what will transpire from one moment to the next (unless, of course, you're ready and willing to put the effort in to achieve the outcome you want.) Rather than physically working toward making something happen, we become stuck in the moment because we are so anxious that things are not going to happen in our favor or in a way that benefits us.

Remember what I said above about how we are the ones who are holding ourselves back? We are the ones who take things that could occur in our lives and flip the switch on them, focusing on our belief that they will occur exactly as we have been fearing this whole time.

This is not to say that what has been a major concern for us from the beginning of a project or assignment will turn out to be nothing. But we set ourselves up for failure just by assuming that the experience we are about to go through will be painful and miserable and one where we are going to be desperately unhappy from start to finish. Despite this being irrational, our minds are unlikely to stop this destructive dialogue with our inner selves. The result is that everything is much harder than it needs to be.

Remember that in the previous chapter, we spoke about how things that appear to be one thing could be something else and that just because you imagine something to be one way doesn't necessarily mean that it is so. Fear has the power to do this to us. It is strong enough to make us believe that the worst outcome is the only outcome to expect.

We also discussed that when we begin to expect something often enough, the universe tends to give it to us. Therefore, expecting only negativity in your life will attract more negativity.

Imagining that something is one way doesn't make it so. Often, it is just a trick of the mind that makes us want to believe that we cannot break out of the mold that fear has us securely fastened to. So how do we unfasten ourselves?

How to Overcome Fear

According to psychologists, a great anagram for the word fear is "fantasized experiences appearing real." This is quite obvious in some cases. Our minds clearly go into hyperdrive, and we psych ourselves up so much that we are often just a hot mess rather than a functioning human being by the end of the process.

Something that is extremely powerful is that because we are the creators of our own fears, we get to control them and even get rid of them.

Two of the ways we can do this that don't take much effort at all are:

- Visualizing
- Controlling where our thoughts go

Fear will consistently play us up against the world, making us out to be the victim of our own circumstances permanently. If we can visualize the threat in front of us or give it some form of a persona, it no longer seems to be so daunting to overcome. Every fear that we have will materialize in some way. If you ask yourself what the worst thing that can happen is, and you find the answer to that, then the fear also begins to lose some of its power.

We are the only ones who are able to control where our thoughts go. I know that there are times when we believe that others have some control over this, but it's simply not true. We can either allow our thoughts to become the most dominant factor in our lives right now, or we can send them off packing because they really have no place to be here.

Some of our thought processes when it comes to fear are still hidden in the subconscious. Before any of this can begin to work, we must be able to get to the point where we are ready to move beyond the subconscious and into the conscious state.

We are the only creatures on Earth with the capacity to make wise decisions concerning our past, present, and future. It's up to us to ensure that all those things that should be left in the past never rear their ugly heads again. While having no fears whatsoever would be living in an ideal environment, we can change our way of thinking from negative to positive instead.

According to Jack Canfield, the master life coach we quoted earlier and a personal development trainer and co-author of most of *The Chicken Soup* books, there is a winning recipe when it comes to making things better for ourselves. The most important parts of this recipe are:

- Creating a list of fears
- Reframing your fears

Let's look at each to see how we can conquer fear once and for all.

Make a List of Your Fears

Complete a comprehensive list of all those things you're too afraid to do. Note that this list is what you are afraid to do, not what you are afraid of. Canfield specifies that there is a difference between things that you are afraid of and things that you are afraid of doing. Consider the following examples.

You suffer from arachnophobia, which is a fear of spiders. This has nothing whatsoever to do with being afraid of speaking in public or approaching management with an idea of how to streamline operations. Can you see how each of these falls into two separate categories? You don't even need to think of different ways to separate these. The first is a fear of something, while the last two are fears of doing something. Keep your list to those that fall in the latter category.

By making a list, you can get to the heart of what is creating the fear for you in the first place. Keep your list as brief as possible, and only include things that you are currently afraid of becoming a reality in your life (Canfield, 2018).

You may choose to include some major life decisions that, up until now, you have been too afraid to face up to. Examples of these could include:

- Leaving your current job and finding another where you earn more money and there are greater opportunities for growth.
- Leaving a long-term relationship that has been hurting your life lately and stunting your growth.

When things like your fears are written down, there's no room for ambiguity. You can clearly see what you are afraid of and what you want to do.

Sitting and writing a list takes a certain degree of discipline and can also help you become more focused on where the problems are. The more time you spend doing this, the more clarity and wisdom you are likely to have to work with and replace each of these fearful tactics. Once you are happy with what you have written down and you believe that you have a complete list, then it's time to begin working on them one by one.

Reframe Your Fears

Once you have identified each of your fears, it is time to begin to reframe them as Canfield proposes. He makes use of the following formula when it comes to putting your fears into sentences that can be made actionable:

I want to __________, and I scare myself by imagining __________.

Take any fear from the list you have written down and try to reframe it using the above sentence to see whether it makes more sense to you. The whole idea behind this process is that you get to take your power back rather than leaving it with your fear. An example of this might read as follows:

I want to *be able to speak in front of people*, but I scare myself by imagining *they will all laugh at me.*

Or

I want to *try running my own business*, but I scare myself by imagining *that it will fail, and I will lose everything.*

Notice how powerful these statements can be. But by changing the narrative, and reframing each of your fears, you can immediately identify exactly what it is that you're afraid of. Once you know what the perceived fear is, you are able to work through it or overcome it. After you have done this, you are going to take the end of the sentence and add something to it that makes you realize that this is exactly the end goal. It needs to be rounded off with something positive that you have passion for, something that's going to make you excited about climbing out of bed in the morning.

Each of your fears should be turned around completely so they now become positive and empowering messages to help you achieve every goal and objective that you set for yourself.

By taking the examples above, we can reframe these fears as follows:

I am confident about speaking in front of people, and even though they may laugh at me, this is not going to stop me from trying my best.

I know that I can run my own business. Yes, there may be risks involved, but I know that if I don't take these risks, I may regret it for the rest of my life.

Working With Fears

There are several ways you can start challenging your fears. Jack Canfield has a number of recommendations that might work for you. This list isn't exhaustive, so if you think of any other techniques, feel free to try them out. Also, keep in mind that some of these may not work for you. That's okay. Keep trying them until you find the ones you like best.

Use Affirmations: Positive affirmations can be found everywhere. You can find affirmations for wealth, health, business, success, relationships, finances, and anything in between. Make your affirmations short, memorable, and always in the present, and hopefully, you will be able to change any negative thought patterns into positive ones.

Some examples of affirmations are:
- I am powerful.

- I can do this.
- I am worthy of love.

Your goal is for you to be able to replace these negative thoughts completely.

Adopt Powerful Emotions: Think of how powerful words and emotions can be together. I have provided an example above of how to reframe some of the thoughts that you have written down in your list of fears. The one thing I haven't mentioned is how powerful words combined with emotions can be. This is one of the reasons for setting up strong positive affirmations using words such as 'happy,' 'positive,' and 'successful.' For example, you could say, "I will be successful." or "I can find happiness." Our words influence our lives far more than we realize or give them credit for.

Avoid Fear-Filled Thoughts: The only way of physically getting this right is by being acutely aware of not only your thoughts but also how each of these thoughts affects you. We have already discussed self-awareness as part of emotional intelligence and being more aware of the emotions that you have. Part of this forms mindfulness techniques where you acknowledge the thought for what it is but you don't hang on to it. This would be especially beneficial whenever your thought patterns are negative or filled with fear. Being able to bring these thoughts and emotions to your awareness allows you to change them. You can do this by choosing positive thoughts and statements to replace the negative ones. Some examples of positive thoughts could include sensations of joy, love, peace, and harmony.

Celebrate Each Win: You do not need to be over the top or have an oversized celebration each time you hit a milestone. But do congratulate yourself when you achieve something you were working toward. Also, it is important to remember the reason why you are doing what you are doing. The interesting thing to mention right here is that most people say that it is not money that motivates them. They find their happiness in other pursuits that are often closely linked with the work that they do. For others, it is the contribution they are able to offer the world without wanting anything in return that motivates them.

Positive Thinking: As mentioned above, it is important for us to realize that we each have the power to get rid of any and all negative thought processes that may be holding us back. This means being able to identify negative thought processes and making our positive thoughts as believable as possible. You can try and change your thoughts as often and as long as you like; however, if you aren't convinced by what you are trying to replace your thought processes with, then you might as well give up. The new thought process must be positive and believable. It must also instill sufficient confidence within you that you can achieve what you are stating you can do. One way to do this would be to take a negative thought, such as "I never do anything right," and challenge it with examples of when you have succeeded. Maybe you aced a test or you gave a killer presentation. Challenge your negative thoughts with those times.

Realism: While we have been talking about a lot of nice characteristics, personality changes, exercises, and techniques that can improve our lives, one of the most important things we need to remember is to be realistic in all that we do. The reason for this is that there is so much fake out there already.

We discussed earlier in this book how using your imagination can only take you so far, and then you need to consider trying to make it on your own. Well, being realistic also helps you to set realistic goals for yourself rather than trying to ride in on someone else's coattails. Yes, it can be to your advantage if you recognize that person for the effort and contributions that have been made toward changing the current situation from one that is fearful and negative to one that's much more positively charged. By using this positive energy, you can try and replace negative energy and sentiments with something that you can believe in. This is why it's so important to ensure that there is positive energy flowing in and all around you.

If you are surrounded by negative energy, focus on positive affirmations, meditation, and shifting your mindset from a negative one to a positive one. There are many tried-and-tested tools that have successfully been used as an intervention whenever fear is present. Remember that fear is just a feeling that is caused by a perception of something. We have covered an extensive list of things that you may find yourself afraid of in the previous chapter.

This chapter will more than likely be your go-to chapter in this book as you work through each of your fears. It is jam-packed with information and ways for you to overcome your fears to get you to move toward the life you'd rather be living. If it feels overwhelming, though, that's okay. Feel free to step back and try one thing at a time. Maybe you start with just making a list of your fears, and then the next week, you start reframing one of them. Progress may be slow, but it will be worth it in the end. With time, you will be able to move forward, which is what we will talk about next.

Chapter 9:

Moving Forward to a Better YOU!

"To help yourself, you must be yourself. Be the best that you can be. When you make a mistake, learn from it, pick yourself up, and move on."
~ Dave Pelzer

There are so many excellent quotes out there about learning those important lessons that life wants you to learn as soon as you possibly can. In the previous chapters, we covered things that are sometimes hard for us to hear. There are many bitter pills that we occasionally need to swallow to progress and grow in our lives. Realize this, though: Somebody has to do it, so why not you?

As many interesting quotes as there are out there, there is also excellent advice from those who have walked this path and been able to change their destiny purely by altering their thought patterns.

How Can You Change Your Thinking?

One of the great masters when it came to introducing positive thinking to the world was author Norman Vincent Peale. He wrote a profound statement, and if we learn how to apply it to our lives, it is certain to change the way we look at everything. He said, "Change your thoughts and you change your world."

Let's analyze this a little bit more and try to take it deeper since we have discovered that learning to silence our inner critic takes more than just trying to put it in the nether regions of our minds. What Peale was trying to get across to each of us is that everything that transpires in our lives boils down to what we choose.

Now, before you start shooting me down for making such a generalized statement, consider this: Good and bad things happen to each of us on a daily basis, right? During the moments following each of these actions, we are faced with something known as a micro-choice or a micro-decision. Most of the time, this is happening on autopilot. Remember how we discussed that the subconscious is in control? This is where the autopilot is steering the ship or flying the plane.

Faced with these tiny micro-decisions, we can either choose to go one way or another. Imagine this process similar to a flow diagram. Someone presents you with two options, A or B, and you need to choose one of them. Going with option A will have one specific outcome attached to it, while going with option B may have something completely different in store for you.

Now, here's where being "wise enough" could potentially save you from being roasted. No matter which of the two options you choose, you need to have the wisdom to stand by your decision and see things through to the end. This is known as responsibility and accountability, and anyone who knows anything about emotional intelligence will be able to tell you that next to integrity, these are two of the most important skills you can ever hope to acquire.

What accountability does in this instance of our flow diagram and decision-making habits is ensure that even when you make the wrong decision, you own it and decide to move forward by choosing something different for yourself. Far too many individuals allow their situation to determine who they are and who they become as a result of their choices, decisions, and actions. Accountability does not allow that. No matter where we are on this journey that is called life, we need to be strong enough to own each decision we make.

You have probably guessed by now that not every choice that we make in life is healthy for us. Many of our decisions are made on the fly, and we are influenced by so many other factors such as:

- Peer pressure
- Material things

- Social media
- Parents
- Employers

In many instances, we are so quick to make a decision that we aren't even aware that one of these micro-decisions presented itself and we switched over to autopilot for our subconscious to choose for us.

Now, I am not saying that every decision we ever make or have made in life needs to be analyzed; however, when we don't get the outcome or result we want, there's always a reason behind it.

Just to prove how powerful and subtle each of these little micro-decisions is, imagine if I implanted in your brain the thought that you are thirsty and need to have something cool to drink to quench your thirst. Before the end of this paragraph, you will probably be thinking about walking over to the refrigerator to see what's cold enough for you to drink!

Just the mere suggestion has made you think about going and getting yourself something cold to drink.

In the section that follows, we are going to focus on how important it is to be able to take accountability and responsibility for your thoughts, words, and actions.

Accountability

One of the strangest parts of accountability is that when things are going right and we've made the right decisions that are leading to success or personal growth or we're achieving the results we're after, we are happy. We don't mind accepting both accountability and responsibility for whatever is happening around us.

It's quite the reverse whenever we make a mistake. When we make a bad decision or something doesn't quite work out the way we wanted it to, then it's not such a comfortable place for us to be in. We tend to point fingers at others and shift blame rather than just owning it and learning how to grow from it instead.

Please understand that as you journey through life, you will never get things right 100% of the time. When you are working with people, there will always be those you get along with and those who, no matter how hard you try, you simply can't gel with. This is part of life. We are each unique with different personalities and characteristics.

Becoming Better Daily

There's an excellent book by James Clear called *Atomic Habits: An Easy & Proven Way to Build Good Habits & Break Bad Ones*. The gist of this book is to strive to do everything in your life just 1% better every day, which we briefly discussed in chapter 4. Is that doable?

Absolutely! He goes on to explain that all those tiny percents will compound over time, and by the end of a specific period, there will be substantial growth in your life. This is much better than trying to do everything all at once (Clear, 2018).

Much like trying to eat an elephant, you do it one small bite at a time. To reach those goals and dreams that you believe are worth chasing, you need to work slowly and consistently toward achieving them. Something that's also worth mentioning at this time is that unfortunately, there are and always will be certain factors that you have no particular control over.

Think about it for a moment. We cannot control things like governments, economies, climate change, or natural disasters. These are going to occur, and we will have little control over these catastrophes. What we can still control, though, is how we respond to each of these situations. We can choose to lie down and stay down, or each time we get knocked down, we can determine where we go in the future.

This can also determine what those inner critics have to say about us. They can either start cheering us on to achieve the things that we have determined to be worthy goals and aspirations, or they can continue to shoot us down. I certainly know which of the two voices I would prefer to listen to.

While we are talking about listening to these voices, something that's important to realize is that we have a choice as to whether we are going to listen to them or replace them with something else.

Agency or Will

This often comes under the guise of many different names—agency, will, freedom to choose, and so on. Each of the micro-decisions that, up until now, we have been making in a subconscious state needs to be brought into our conscious state. How do we manage to get that right, though? There are so many things going on in our heads, especially on a subconscious level that you may not have even realized you were doing this—till now. That's why you need to STOP.

STOP

I was listening to a podcast several years ago that was about judging others, but I believe that some of the content can be applied here because there's an important lesson to be learned about our thought processes and how we perceive those around us. Instead of constantly sitting in judgment of those around us, why don't we focus inward instead? Instead of focusing on others, let's focus on ourselves and our own subconscious.

Having the freedom to act, react, or respond to situations as they are presented to us daily is something we don't always bring into our conscious mind. This is what we need to do so that each of our decisions, choices, and actions ends up being the best we are able to do at the time.

Earlier in this book, I spoke about us sleepwalking through life, where we don't pay much attention to whatever is happening around us. This is one of the micro-decisions we need to STOP. We need to accept responsibility and accountability for the way we behave in our lives, and we need to STOP pointing fingers at everyone else. Just because others don't do things the same way that we do doesn't mean that their way is necessarily wrong. It means that their way is different. Differences should be celebrated, not frowned upon.

Can you imagine how boring life and this world would be if we all looked the same, had the same taste in clothing and fashion, had the same opinions about food and drinks, and had the same taste in companions?

Focus on accepting and celebrating the differences in humanity, cultures, global traditions, and even within your own home and family. Consider ways that you can assume full responsibility for your life and every aspect of it.

This poem by Sivananda may put the microcosm into perspective for you:

> A mountain is composed of tiny grains of earth. The ocean is made up of tiny drops of water. Even so, life is but an endless series of little details, actions, speeches, and thoughts. And the

consequences whether good or bad of even the least of them are far-reaching.

We need to stop and consider each of the minute details in our lives because compounded, they add up to big things.

Changes to Your Lifestyle

You were specifically drawn to this book because either there is something about your life at the moment that you're not happy with or because you're trying to quiet the excessive chatter that's constantly going on in your head. One of the ways you can do this successfully is by making small, incremental changes to your lifestyle. Each of these choices will compound and result in something substantial over time.

Several years ago, there was a challenge that was making the rounds that started with just one push-up. It was a limited daily challenge where you had to add a push-up for each day you were participating. Now, you may be thinking to yourself, what's the big deal with this type of challenge, especially for someone who is already fit?

The challenge wasn't so much one of getting fit; that was a by-product of regular participation in the challenge. The main goal of the challenge was to get you into a specific routine of being able to do something. It was teaching the valuable lesson of forming habits.

There's some debate as to whether it takes 21 days to form a habit, or whether it takes 30 to 60 days to ensure that a habit is firmly entrenched and part of your psyche. Regardless, the moment you choose to become fully committed to doing something, come rain, hail, sleet, or snow, then you know that you are changing your lifestyle for the better.

It's not my place to tell you that you need to implement a fitness regime or make changes to your eating habits as part of staying physically fit. You may be 100% sorted in each of these areas; however, maybe the area that you need to be working on is meditation. Or you may need to sharpen your mindfulness techniques as a way to tone down the voices of each of your internal critics.

The rest of this chapter is going to be dedicated to some ideas that you may want to start implementing in your life in small and simple ways on a daily, weekly, or monthly basis.

Let's look at breaking some of these lifestyle habits down into workable groups. Should you feel that there are certain groups that don't fit you, feel free to skip over them until you come across one that resonates with you. Once you can identify one that will change your life, even in a small way at first, start implementing those particular habits.

Before we begin, remember that there are probably going to be days when you make mistakes and you skip a day. Rather than throwing your hands in the air, proclaiming that it's no good, or you're a failure (sounding like your inner critic?), simply pick up again on the next day, and try not to be too hard on yourself. These are incremental changes that you are adding to your existing lifestyle.

Lifestyle Habits

Health and Fitness: If you don't have an exercise program in place, then begin one. It doesn't matter if you decide to start with a single push-up challenge or walking for five minutes in your neighborhood. The ideal scenario would be to start slowly, especially if you aren't currently doing anything to keep your body physically fit. Part of this may also include making reasonable changes to your diet. Maybe it's the way you prepare your meals or cutting back on all the junk foods you eat. Once you get into it, you will find that there are a lot of changes in this area of your life that you can begin implementing.

Finances: Are you currently following a budget? Do you know where the bulk of your financial spending is going each month? Do you have a savings plan? Are you able to set aside a certain amount of money toward sound financial investments? How can you trim your budget each month? Do you have too much money left at the end of the month? Have you met with a financial planner? Are your taxes up to date? All of these are questions to consider when looking at your financial habits.

Meditation: This could cover several different aspects of your life between your physical, spiritual, and emotional well-being. Meditation can take on a wealth of different formats, and you don't need to be stuck in any particular one. Some people prefer to meditate in silence or in prayer, while others prefer reading scripture. And still, others practice yoga, tai chi, and other Asian-inspired activities. For others, Pilates can help them refocus and strengthen their core muscles.

With meditation, there is no singular activity that is either correct or incorrect. The most important aspect is that it needs to be something that you are comfortable with. Whether that means ringing Tibetan bowls first thing in the morning or writing in a journal, the main benefit comes from having some quiet alone time with your thoughts where you are able to process where you are and where you can gain the maximum benefit. One of the main benefits of meditation is that you get in touch with who you are as an individual inwardly.

Physically: This not only covers things like your actual physical appearance, the way you dress, and the way you carry yourself, but it also covers how you take care of your body in general. Are you getting sufficient rest at night? Do you visit your doctor for regular check-ups whenever they are due? Are you using wisdom when it comes to what you're putting into your body? Even simple things such as hydration count. Are you making sure that you drink enough water during the day? Do you take care of your skin, hair, and nails? If you suffer from any form of vitamin or mineral deficiencies, are you currently taking any supplements to counteract this?

Mentally: There's a quotation by Albert Einstein that says that anyone can be a genius in any subject if they study the actual subject for just 15 minutes each day! This alone can tell us a bit more about the mental capacity that we have available to us. Do we make the best use of this capacity, or are we happy to allow it to stagnate by feeding it garbage? While this may sound a bit harsh, let's tell it like it is. When you feed your mind, brain, or intellect absolute trash, then don't be surprised when this is exactly what you are going to get back. Things that you could be feeding your beautiful mind and intellect are things like personal development, self-help, and motivational material. This book is a great place to start. That doesn't mean you have to toss out the romance novel, but try to incorporate some things that will build you up.

Career: Set specific career goals for yourself as to where you see yourself in five years. If that feels like a lot, you can pull it back to three years, then again to one year, and even six months. While it's fine to have these goals set in place, how do you plan to get there? Find yourself a mentor or someone that you admire who's in a more senior role. Use them as a sounding board to help you accomplish all of your career aspirations.

Relationships: What do you want to achieve from your relationships? This could be anything from your relationship with your spouse, partner, or significant other. It could even be your relationship with your children or other family members. It's important that you figure out how to work with and get along with people from all walks of life. We've already mentioned that we are all different, and we celebrate the fact that we are unique humans, each here having a different experience called life.

Education: The day you stop learning is the day you die. We should each push ourselves further every day. If you set a goal that you will learn at least one new thing each day, consider that this alone compounded over a year will lead to at least 365 new things learned over the year. You can also consider a formal education. There are more and more senior citizens, baby boomers, and those of the silent generation who are making it their mission to still keep their minds active. This doesn't have to be expensive, though. There are plenty of low-cost options online, and some are even free.

Journal: Get into the habit of keeping a journal; even a short and sweet bullet journal will work where you can record your highs and lows for the day. You will be amazed by the amount of growth you can recognize in yourself and those around you simply by going through the journals at a later stage. There will also potentially be a lot of important information from your life that you may want to remember late. This could indicate growth in your children through childhood and adolescence. It's amazing the intuitive nature they have, which shines through years later as you go through these records.

You can also keep a gratitude journal. This is similar to a normal journal, but it is just a quick couple of notes that express what you've been grateful for on that particular day. The idea behind it is to just list three to five things that you are grateful for throughout the day. Try not to write the same thing every day, of course. You may be surprised by how many things you have to be grateful for.

Forcing your mind to look for things to be grateful for also gives you the opportunity of shifting your focus from your inner critics to more positive thinking, which will help to reduce the volume of your inner critics.

You will be able to find examples of each of these journals online or physically at most reputable bookstores. In addition to these, there are even apps that you can download from both the Google Play and Apple stores. The beauty of choosing to work with apps on your mobile device is that you can set reminders to complete these specific tasks at a preselected time of the day.

Rest and Relaxation: This is something we all need to be able to enjoy. For those who are addicted to work, this is especially for you. Please understand that you are not meant to be pushing all the boundaries when it comes to mental stimulation and trying to have your finger on the pulse of too many things simultaneously. It's going to lead to burnout, and then what?

Some of the best advice I have ever received is something I would like to share with you as this book comes to a close. "All things in moderation can be a good thing." I give credit to the author anonymously.

The reason for focusing on each of these areas individually is so that you can see that your goals, hopes, dreams, desires, and aspirations need to be evenly spaced and well balanced. By keeping each of these areas in balance, your life itself will be kept balanced. A balanced life is a happy one.

It can sometimes be hard to see how beautiful life is, especially when we are focused on the negative.

There have been many tips, tools, and strategies shared with you in the last few pages of this book. This is by no means an exhaustive list of some of the things that you could be doing. Instead, these things are meant to help you get started. They are here to give you a bit of a springboard toward your future. A future that is more organized, one that is fully focused on you being able to extract the maximum benefit from life.

It's my desire that you try and implement as many of these into your daily life as you possibly can. Within a short time, the compounding effect that is spoken of by James Clear in *Atomic Habits* will start to occur. It worked for me, and it can work for everyone. I'm not going to dictate where you start. You know where you need these changes most in your life.

Getting back to your harsh inner critics. One of the best ways to get rid of them is by learning how to replace them with other voices. This is where journaling is able to help you identify those times in your life when things were maybe simpler, and you were achieving everything you set your mind to. You need to send your present-day mentality back to this point. Mentally, you need to be able to recognize that you have succeeded at similar things before, and you can probably easily repeat the process.

Turn the volume down using mindfulness exercises. Try and identify each individual voice that forms part of your inner critic. Remember that you don't necessarily have to be listening to any of these. After all, they are the direct result of a much earlier time in your life. Do the things that they have to say have validity now? Chances are that they don't. Challenge them the way we talked about earlier.

Use your own wisdom when choosing which of these voices you are going to allow to impact your life. It is my sincere wish for you that the only voices you pay attention to moving forward are those voices that are going to positively influence you. Be sure to get out there and live your best life possible!

As an author, it is my job to ensure that I always deliver the highest-quality product possible with information that is relevant to the material. If you have enjoyed this book, please consider leaving a comment on Amazon to let me know. I would love to see how you have freed yourself from your inner critics.

References

A-Z Quotes. (n.d.). *Top 25 limiting beliefs quotes.* A-Z Quotes. Retrieved February 9, 2021, from https://www.azquotes.com/quotes/topics/limiting-beliefs.html

Alvarez, E. (2020, May 20). *How to stop listening to your inner critic.* Medium. https://medium.com/@emily_alvarez/how-to-stop-listening-to-your-inner-critic-f2b39fe9aa54

Amatenstein, S. (2016). *Facing your fears: Tips to overcoming anxiety and phobias.* Psycom.net - Mental Health Treatment Resource since 1986. https://www.psycom.net/facing-your-fear

Blackman, A. (2018, August 11). *What are self-limiting beliefs? +How to overcome them successfully.* Business Envato Tuts+. https://business.tutsplus.com/tutorials/what-are-self-limiting-beliefs--cms-31607

Bundrant, M. (2012, December 18). *How to overcome limiting beliefs that hold you back from success.* Lifehack. https://www.lifehack.org/articles/productivity

/stop-limiting-beliefs-and-take-back-your-life.html

Byrne, R. (2016). *The secret: the 10th anniversary edition*. Atria Books; Hillsboro, Or. (Original work published 2006)

Canfield, J. (2018, April 25). *Overcoming fear: How to realize fear is created by you | Jack Canfield*. Jackcanfield. https://www.jackcanfield.com/blog/overcoming-fear/

Chierotti, L. (2018, April 27). *Is fear stopping you from achieving your goals? Overcome it by understanding these 3 principles*. Inc.com. https://www.inc.com/logan-chierotti/is-fear-stopping-you-from-achieving-your-goals-overcome-it-by-understanding-these-3-principles.html

Clear, J. (2018). *Atomic habits: tiny changes, remarkable results: an easy & proven way to build good habits & break bad ones*. Avery, An Imprint Of Penguin Random House.

Firestone, L. (2013, May 14). *4 Ways to overcome your inner critic*. Psychology Today. https://www.psychologytoday.com/za/blog/compassion-matters/201305/4-ways-overcome-your-inner-critic

Fishel, B. (2019, January 12). *24 Quotes about moving on and forward thinking*. KeepInspiring.me. https://www.keepinspiring.me/24-quotes-moving-on-forward-thinking/

Gary John Bishop. (2017). *Unf*ck yourself get out of your head and into your life*. London Yellow Kite.

Goodreads. (n.d.). *Inner critic quotes (25 quotes)*. Www.goodreads.com. Retrieved February 10, 2021, from https://www.goodreads.com/quotes/tag/inner-critic

Johnstone, D. (2019, July 22). *9 Self limiting beliefs that are holding you back from success*. Lifehack. https://www.lifehack.org/839222/self-limiting

Leggett, T. J. (2019, November 8). *Ruminating thoughts: How to stop them*. Www.medicalnewstoday.com. https://www.medicalnewstoday.com/articles/326944

Lipton, B. H. (2016). *The biology of belief: unleashing the power of consciousness, matter & miracles*. Hay House, Inc. (Original work published 2005)

Manson, M. (2020, November 12). *How to overcome your limiting beliefs*. Mark Manson. https://markmanson.net/limiting-beliefs/

Morin, A. (2014, November 6). *Taming your inner critic: 7 Steps to silencing the negativity.* Forbes. https://www.forbes.com/sites/amymorin/201 4/11/06/taming-your-inner-critic-7-steps-to-silencing-the-negativity/

Morin, A. (2018, September 14). *3 Types of self-limiting beliefs that will keep you stuck in life (and what to do about them).* Inc.com. https://www.inc.com/amy-morin/3-types-of-unhealthy-beliefs-that-will-drain-your-mental-strength-make-you-less-effective.html

Newman, L. (2011, July 5). *5 Immediate and easy ways to silence your inner critic.* Tiny Buddha. https://tinybuddha.com/blog/5-immediate-and-easy-ways-to-silence-your-inner-critic/

Pincott, J. E. (2019). *Silencing your inner critic.* Psychology Today. https://www.psychologytoday.com/us/articles /201903/silencing-your-inner-critic

Real Life Counseling. (2018, June 21). *6 Strategies to overcome fear and anxiety.* Real Life Counseling. https://reallifecounseling.us/overcome-fear-and-anxiety/0

Roomer, J. (2018, December 13). *4 Fears that are stopping you from achieving your best life (and how to overcome it).* Medium. https://medium.com/personal-growth-lab/4-fears-that-are-stopping-you-from-achieving-

your-best-life-and-how-to-overcome-it-
67c7f5950e5a#

SARK. (1991). *A creative companion: how to free your creative spirit.* Celestial Arts.

Sasson, R. (2017, July 15). *How to live a positive lifestyle.* Success Consciousness. https://www.successconsciousness.com/blog/positive-attitude/how-to-live-a-positive-lifestyle/

Savage, R. (2020, February 3). *How to overcome your own self-limiting beliefs.* Medium. https://medium.com/better-humans/how-to-overcome-your-own-self-limiting-beliefs-6bb517dc8d73

Schaffner, K. (2020, October 15). *Living with your inner critic: 8 Helpful worksheets and activities.* PositivePsychology.com. https://positivepsychology.com/inner-critic-worksheets/

Sims Wyeth. (2014, October 10). *17 Inspiring quotes to help you face your fears.* Inc.com; Inc. https://www.inc.com/sims-wyeth/17-inspiring-quotes-to-help-you-face-your-fears.html

Smith, A. K. (2017). *The bravest you: five steps to fight your biggest fears, find your passion, and unlock your extraordinary life.* Tarcherperigee.

Snyder, B. (2017, May 18). *The 10 biggest fears holding you back from success.* CNBC; CNBC. https://www.cnbc.com/2017/05/18/the-10-biggest-fears-holding-you-back-from-success.html

Steimle, J. (2016, January 4). *14 Ways to conquer fear.* Forbes. https://www.forbes.com/sites/joshsteimle/2016/01/04/14-ways-to-conquer-fear/

SUCCESS Staff. (2017, October 26). *15 Quotes to overcome your self-limiting beliefs.* SUCCESS. https://www.success.com/15-quotes-to-overcome-your-self-limiting-beliefs/

teamuapeaknet. (2020, January 5). *The inner critic—your biggest obstacle to happiness.* Peak. https://blog.peak.net/2020/01/05/the-inner-critic/

Tet. (n.d.). *55 Quotes on overcoming fear.* Productive and Free. https://www.productiveandfree.com/blog/overcoming-fear-quotes

Thibodeaux, W. (2018, May 21). *Why you might not want to silence your inner critic completely, according to psychology.* Inc.com. https://www.inc.com/wanda-thibodeaux/why-you-might-not-want-to-silence-your-inner-critic-completely-according-to-psychology.html

Tracy, B. (2017, March 27). *How to overcome your fears, get unstuck, and fuel your success |...* Brian Tracy's Self Improvement & Professional Development Blog. https://www.briantracy.com/blog/personal-success/fight-or-flight-overcoming-your-fears/

Virgo, J. (2015, August 24). *Understanding your inner critic.* The Everygirl. https://theeverygirl.com/understanding-your-inner-critic/

Whitener, S. (2020, June 26). How to use empowering beliefs to overcome limiting beliefs and find freedom. *Forbes.* https://www.forbes.com/sites/forbescoachescouncil/2020/06/25/how-to-use-empowering-beliefs-to-overcome-limiting-beliefs-and-find-freedom/

Williams, J. V. M. (2019). *Goodbye me hello me: Letting go of the past, to embrace your future.* Ad libris.